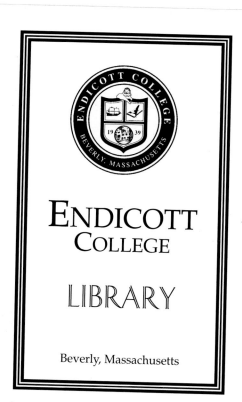

SHATTERED MIRRORS

SHATTERED *Mirrors*

Our Search for Identity and Community in the AIDS Era

Monroe E. Price

Harvard University Press
Cambridge, Massachusetts
London, England   1989

This book is printed on acid-free paper, and its binding materials
have been chosen for strength and durability.

Library of Congress Cataloging-in-Publication Data

Price, Monroe Edwin, 1938–
   Shattered mirrors : our search for identity and community in the
   AIDS era / Monroe E. Price.
     p. cm.
   Bibliography: p.
   Includes index.
   ISBN 0-674-80590-9 (alk. paper)
   1. AIDS (Disease)—Social aspects—United States. I. Title.
RA644.A25P755 1989   89-33265
306.4'61—dc20   CIP

For Aimée

Contents

Prologue

It is, even now, early in the crisis that is AIDS, but the pressures on our society and on our attitudes toward basic rights and freedoms are mounting. The challenge to the public's health is creating a faultline beneath our institutions, threatening to undermine much that we have taken for granted about the pillars of our culture. We look out across the landscape of AIDS and see not merely a change here or there but a fundamental rearrangement in the way we think about ourselves and about others. We sense a silent shuddering adjustment, the combination of millions of private recognitions of a shifting context. Not just our intimate relationships but also our concept of citizenship is suddenly vulnerable.

Some events have extraordinary immediate impact but do not, in the long run, alter our social institutions nor the ideals by which people live. Other events leave an indelible mark on the life of the community. Initially, AIDS seemed to be of the former order, a plague in slow motion, as Richard Goldstein has called it, strangely circumscribed, a disease of them and not of us.[1] It is only a matter of time, we told ourselves, until this disease, like so many others, is scientifically described, its workings ascertained, its capacity to cause death conquered.

These thoughts of closure, comfortable to have, proved wanting. As the number of infected people mounted, even as early hopes for an instant cure or vaccine receded into the distance, government and the media undertook the struggle to redefine

AIDS, to reconceive the disease as one that affects us all. In the hands of the image-makers, AIDS became a moral lesson for our nation—not about the dangers of deviancy but about the personal responsibility that comes with freedom.

Yet the seemingly straightforward task of teaching individual accountability has troubling ramifications that bore deeper into the structure of our society than exhortations to practice safe sex and abjure drugs might suggest; for it is through strong government intervention that individual accountability—the basic building block in our defense against AIDS—is being created. To seize the moment for public instruction, government has forcefully asserted a set of values that is at odds with much our culture teaches. Yet in the face of crisis we have been inclined to suspend doubts about government's rightful role in reshaping the ideals and images of our time. We have witnessed the reemergence of alliances of morality in a closer bonding between church and state, as religious institutions have sought to influence the words and acts of public health officials in devising their strategies. The media, too, have felt the sting of urgency to revise the images they promote, in order to conform to the public health messages of the state. Here, then, may be one of the hardest legacies of AIDS: that it has forced us to recalculate the cost of protecting private values and decisions from the power and domain of government influence.

At the beginning of its first decade, AIDS was perceived as the gay plague. Under the influence of government, the press, and our own individual fears, it has been transformed into a disease that preoccupies us all. Yet as we move, now, from the first to the second decade of AIDS, our sense of the disease is changing markedly once again. The demography of AIDS—the profile of new cases, the austere tables that weekly report the awesome progress of the disease—shows that AIDS is becoming more and more a plague of the urban poor, the neglected underclass. In some major cities, 1 in 60 newborns is infected with AIDS; in poverty-stricken areas where drug use is high, the figure may be 1 baby in 45. AIDS is rending the already tenuous fabric of life among poor blacks and Hispanics in city ghettos.

As the face of AIDS becomes transfigured in its second decade, so will our response as a society. The danger is that preoccupation with the epidemic will diminish because of general disdain for problems of the poor or because of an ill-founded belief that the wall between the urban poor and the rest of society is less permeable than the wall between those who are bisexual or gay and those who are not. As fear recedes, the pressure for public education is likely to diminish as well. AIDS may once again become less about the conduct of all of us and more about public policy toward an already submerged class, one that is largely minority and largely outside the sympathies of the wider society.

In other places, other times, overwhelming fear of a fatal, contagious disease has been a dominating force in changing the nature of the state. Against the backdrop of medieval plague, the growth of local governments can be seen as the rise of public responsibility for the health of citizens. In times of mass infection, the state and its agents become charged with setting limits on public assembly, with establishing dwelling houses for the sick, and with developing strategies for isolating stricken households. But measures to protect the public's health, however empirical their basis, always reflect some of the biases of those in power. Of his experience with nineteenth-century cholera in England, one public health officer wrote: "On several occasions, when disease became excessive, and the men in power and the better classes in general became alarmed for their own safety, they gave some attention to the undrained and filthy conditions of the localities and the abodes of the lower classes, and made some temporary efforts to remove the evils; but that no sooner had the impressive period of danger passed over them than the drainage and cleansing were neglected as before."[2]

In the United States, AIDS is not of the dimensions of medieval plague. But it has devastatingly struck a finely tuned society whose members have high expectations that technology, coupled with government, can provide adequate assurance about the future. AIDS is becoming a watershed of our time because it is shaking our confidence in the ability of bureaucrats and experts to cope with unexpected challenges. AIDS is disruptive because of the agonizing fear it engenders that the course of life is suddenly without its expected control, whether by the individual, by government, or by medicine and science.

As with any epidemic of great magnitude, we learn from AIDS that disease is not just a set of facts but a collection of ideas about the culture, ideas that have a power of their own. The "true" meaning of AIDS eludes us, though we seek to shape that meaning at every turn. No one can foresee how the microorganisms themselves will change and adjust, just as no one can satisfactorily explain why the epidemiological patterns in the United States could be so different from those in parts of Africa, where AIDS occurs predominantly among heterosexuals. So long as we are uncertain about the future course of the disease, we will continue to debate the meaning of AIDS, what an appropriate response to the crisis must be, and how the disease will contribute to shaping our society's image of itself.

We think of AIDS primarily as infiltrating personal relationships, but AIDS is beginning to permeate our arts and letters, jobs and housing, the functioning of the criminal justice system, the structure of insurance coverage, the profile of medical careers, the way we screen the blood supply, develop drugs, care for the terminally ill. Scores of new social, legal, and medical problems have arisen with the AIDS epidemic, and thus far we have reached remarkably few solutions.

Nevertheless, for many of us, AIDS is becoming internalized, as just another threatening fact of life, like the possibility of earthquake or nuclear war—in the background of consciousness but not a disruption of the rhythm of everyday life. Yet this epidemic may have enduring consequences for our future. Already the potential is becoming apparent—how this disease might alter the value we place on individual freedom of expression and freedom from government intervention; how it might change our view of fairness, equal treatment under the law, and discrimination; how it might call into question modern ideas of science and progress, and revive an ancient awareness of vulnerability and death. As AIDS shatters, one by one, the cultural mirrors that have defined our relationships and ourselves since the 1960s, this epidemic may force us, finally, to reconsider what we mean by identity and community in a democracy under siege.

part one

AIDS *and Free Expression*

I do my thing, and you do your thing.
I am not in this world to live up to your expectations.
And you are not in this world to live up to mine.
You are you and I am I,
And if by chance we find each other, it's beautiful.
If not, it can't be helped.

Frederick S. Perls, *Gestalt Therapy Verbatim*, 1969

one

Sexual Imagery and the Media

AIDS strikes at the heart of the most intimate of human relationships, sexual closeness. In so doing, it has fractured what had become the basis of a new social identity. Not for everyone, but for a significant number in our society, the search for sexual fulfillment, the wonder of new partners, the thrill of spontaneous, unrestrained, luxurious lovemaking—these have been among the central motivations of our time, permeating music, television, advertising, motion pictures, theater, and literature.

Here was the idea of freedom rendered available, satisfying, concrete. Far more than a way of selling movie tickets or travel to the Mediterranean, the idea of sexual freedom has been, for the generations that have come of age since the 1960s, synonymous with freedom itself, with a sense of individual possibility, a powerful metaphor for the way we define ourselves and our capabilities. We assert sexual freedom virtually as a badge of the openness and creativity of our society, as a fulfillment of some unarticulated constitutional promise of individual autonomy.

This may seem like a great exaggeration, but only if it is taken as a description of the actual conduct of men and women. The millions who watch soap operas do not necessarily replicate— or even think they will replicate—the conduct they see there. But they do define themselves as living in a society where the conduct they witness is possible. Even if they recognize that what is being performed is religiously or morally forbidden, they see it legitimated to the extent that it unfurls unencumbered on the living room screen. And whether or not sexual liberation, as it is often called, is realized in the daily sex life of the majority, as an ideal it has had immense implications for family structure, for attitudes toward work and leisure, indeed for the shaping, even architecture, of cities. The ideal of liberation has affected decisions about where to live, if and when to marry, whether to have children, whether to divorce.

The celebration of individuality and personal autonomy that is so inextricably wrapped up in our images of sexual freedom—all this has been put at risk by the AIDS epidemic. The symbols of sexuality that permeate our culture have become inconsistent with the public health need for a very different basis upon which to establish our sense of self-fulfillment. Sexual autonomy is rapidly being transformed from a sign of individual freedom into a source of potential death. The emergence of sexual autonomy as a powerful national symbol in the 1960s changed the national consciousness for three decades; a change in symbolism, driven by the pressing public health needs of the 1990s, could alter our sense of self for the foreseeable future.

The process of change in the national consciousness—and therefore in public imagery—is taking place gradually, but noticeably. It is an arresting combination of the voluntary actions of those who guide media, the forces of economics, and the subtle pressures of government and public opinion. Already, motion picture scripts are being rewritten and records are being censored more stringently by radio stations. Television plots that would have been selected are now being rejected, and the images that have come to dominate advertising are changing as well. Industries that for years have been fending off external demands for censorship now fitfully but quite palpably are altering the visage of American entertainment. It is too early to determine how extensive and how rapid these changes will be, just as it is too early to know how threatening the AIDS crisis will ultimately become. But even at present levels of fear, those who are the gatekeepers and image makers of the culture have become increasingly conscious of the fact that a change must come, that those whose work has such a significant impact on the way people live must act to benefit the public health effort.

They realize that in the long absence of any vaccine, they cannot celebrate the older, freer ways, at least so long as personal caution in sexual conduct seems to be the most important way of controlling the spread of AIDS. They know too well that casual attitudes toward personal relations have been deeply reinforced through the media, and that, if these attitudes are to be altered, a sweeping revolution in the way the media depict sexual behavior may be necessary. This recognition has come not through imposition of new laws or government regulation but through a self-originated sense of the mood and need of the country, from what is left of a feeling of communal responsibility, and, undoubtedly, from the personal pain and loss within the entertainment industry, resulting from the death and dying of friends.

The assumption that the media have a substantial impact on conduct and attitudes has a long tradition. The money spent on advertising is ample testimony to the faith of American enterprise in this proposition. Believing in the power of the media over cultural values, underrepresented and outsider groups have tried to affect the way they are reflected in television shows and commercials, in textbooks, and in other mirrors of ourselves. They have tried to correct perceived abuses, such as the absence of minorities and the elderly on television shows, or the depiction of Italians as gangsters, or gangsters as Italians. At first, these efforts tended to be private in nature, conducted by civic groups in conversations behind closed doors with those who shape popular images. More recently, methods for bringing about change in the media have become increasingly public and sophisticated: threats of government regulation or boycotts of products or productions. In the process, law and regulation have become a way to enshrine a vision of a democratic society, as opposed merely to a means of incorporating and reflecting realities. These pressures on the media are intense, because

those groups that want to refashion attitudes and conduct recognize that it is easier to change them through the shaping of
images than to do so directly. Thus, groups with a social agenda
of this kind seek to have the media alter the public's perception
so as to prepare the audience for a romanticized future by in-
sinuating that it already exists.

If we view television, for example, as a medium of social
realism that teaches us who we are and, more interesting, who
we should be, then the efforts by racial minorities, by women,
by business interests, by the handicapped to revise that pro-
jected image are more understandable. Television is not alone.
Twenty years ago, Adam Clayton Powell held hearings on the
way in which minorities, particularly African-Americans, were
depicted in school textbooks. Despite their discomfort, publishers came before his committee to help it evaluate whether a
proper function of government was to question the content of
material taught widely in public schools. For Powell, the answer
was obvious: What people read in textbooks about themselves
and others helps to define their identity. Impatiently, he was
asking whether history, to the extent it can be accurate at all,
was being distorted—distorted in a discriminatory way in the
"official" material young people read—and whether a particular
representation of history and the role of minorities would ben-
eficially influence civic attitudes in the future.[1]

In the two decades since Powell's hearings, the debate about
the role of government in holding the media, including the
publishers of textbooks, accountable for the way in which they
portray and affect segments of the society has become virtually
institutionalized. Not only African-Americans and other racial
minorities but women, the elderly, and advocates for children
all have come to the table asking the same questions: Are you
harming us by the way you are depicting us? Are we becoming
who you say we are? Does the power of your message strongly
influence the struggle for identity within each of us?

With the coming of the AIDS crisis, these kinds of inquiries
and demands are more generalized, pitched at the overall im-

pact of television and the media on society as a whole, not at the relationship between a particular segment and the entirety. Suddenly, the concern is with the way the *mainstream* is portrayed, a concern growing not from the rancor of discrimination but from fear. To be sure, strong vestiges of the minority agenda and perspective still abound: for example, in increased worry about the depiction of homosexuals and the potential for isolation and rancor that could flow from false and condemnatory stereotyping. But the issue becomes much broader: how individuals are portrayed in modern life, what their values are and should be, what conduct will be deemed worthy of imitation, and, as a result, how behavior will be shaped. Not out of a political agenda, nor a utopian vision for the future, but rather out of intense worry about survival, these issues arise and assault one of the central themes of modern life and art, namely, how the society defines the relationship between men and women. And because the anxiety is so widespread and the question so pervasive in its implications, the response has been immediate. Even without government regulation, the media have changed.

Exactly how this process of change is taking place varies from industry to industry. Each area of expression plays a different role in shaping our sense of personal identity, and each has a different relationship to government. What is often called the gatekeeping function—the ability of arbiters of taste to determine the content of the message—is also different for each industry. So is the nature of the audience, how old or young it is, how publicly or privately it enjoys the medium. All of these factors contribute to an understanding of how each medium has developed, how it contributes to ideas about personal liberties and sexual autonomy, and how it is affected by the AIDS crises.

The Balcony as Classroom

Almost from the start, the motion picture industry has been a merchant of romance, and the balcony, or its modern counterpart, has been a place to escape. The handsome leading men and ravishing leading ladies who virtually defined the genre during the twenties and thirties may have, from time to time, played the role of the girl or boy next door, but they remained nevertheless remote and inaccessible. One could aspire to be like them, in the way one held a cigarette, or cocked one's head, or wore a hat, but the reach was great, the distance forbidding.

Motion pictures in recent decades have been a different story. Joan Crawford gave way to Audrey Hepburn, who gave way in turn to Annette Funicello and, ultimately, to Rosanna Arquette. Movies now portray, to a far greater extent, the real people next door, people much like the audience except that these ordinary people somehow manage to lead exciting lives. Instead of stimulating its audience to merely imitate certain affectations of film stars—in the way one might emulate royalty—movies in recent years have seemed to provoke their audience into asking why their own lives are not as charged as the lives of the otherwise very similar people depicted on the screen. At the dawn of the AIDS epidemic, the movies had become less of an escape, more of an immediate prescription for a change of lifestyle.

This transformation in the role of films as teachers or molders of behavior has been inextricably tied to a demographic transformation in the market. As television ate away at the previously massive adult audience of motion pictures, teenagers—with their restless urge to get out of the house and congregate with peers—became the single most important target of the film industry. In the 1970s and 1980s a special conversation between the industry and its audience was established, one that recognized the rebelliousness of youth and spoke the language of dissent. It was on the large screen, not its smaller cousin, that Cheech and Chong could flaunt marijuana as a symbol of liberation. Movies such as *Easy Rider* became the medium of the antihero. The path of the young rebel first pioneered on the screen by James Dean and Marlon Brando had, for teenage America, become the middle of the road.

A crucial element in this new consciousness, and in this commercially successful dialogue between Hollywood and the young, was the bold assertion of sexual autonomy—the liberation of the young, and women in particular, from the sexual mores of their parents. Much of the strength of the film industry in the last two decades was built on the importance to those in the demographic target of this rich and important dialogue about sexual behavior.

The film industry's new intimacy with its young audience was established at a time when fewer and fewer curbs were being imposed by individuals or custom, and virtually none by government, on the way that sexual relations could be depicted on the silver screen. Film producers have not had to deal with the dilemma facing producers for network television that at some level the government affects the medium of exhibition, through its ability to grant or withhold licenses. Compared with television, the film production business is fairly easy to enter. The ability to produce an independent film and have it screened requires money and distribution, of course, but government approval in the form of a license is not necessary.

Motion pictures do not have to enter the living room war fought both by parents and children and by networks alike over the family identity. Television has to meet several sets of standards all at once; many would argue that it meets none of them very well. A movie is a much more private affair, targeted to the tastes and values of its particular audience. Even when movies are invited into the home, in the form of video cassettes, the impact has been only to enhance the privateness of films. VCRs allow the individual to establish, free of coercion, the set of messages that will be reinforced, the company that he or she will keep while receiving them, and even the time of day or night that the viewing will take place.

If the halcyon days of Hollywood still existed, the executives of the small number of studios who controlled production might collusively set standards of taste. But given the high degree of competition in production and among the various methods of exhibition, the likelihood of the industry's agreeing to restrain itself is quite low. In that sense, the film industry is remarkably democratic. No agency determines the way in which any particular film affects either the health of the industry or the health of the nation.

The evolution of the industry-imposed classification and rating system captures this loose relationship between industry structure, gatekeeping, and self-censorship. During the Hays Code, commencing in 1930, the rules about what could be shown and what could not were quite detailed and comprehensive. By contrast, under the current ratings program, administered by the Motion Picture Association of America, there are no effective prohibitions; the idea, rather, is to inform. The primary barrier is an X or R rating, but only the X rating is a significant obstacle, for only it means that a picture cannot gain wide distribution. The rules for PG13, the most common rating, have steadily changed since the introduction of the rating system. This ranking, which sets only a guideline for parental supervision, deals primarily with particular sorts of explicit sexual behavior but does not prohibit the portrayal of attitudes inconsistent with concerns about preventing AIDS. PG13 films have regularly shown practices and attitudes which public health programs are now desperately trying to alter.

Success at the box office has always turned on the ability of a film's promoters to persuade a modern audience that the film at least touches, usually confirms, and perhaps expands, their fantasies. In the decade before AIDS, this meant the portrayal of attitudes that are now, as physicians would say, contraindicated. In the age of AIDS, the movie industry is at least playing with a new consciousness. During the making of a motion picture called *Casual Sex?* the producers debated the issue of whether a question mark should go in the title. Without the question mark, the producers worried about the mild advocacy, the suggestion that this is more of the pre-AIDS culture. With the question mark, the movie asks the question that is on the minds of its audience: What can be done? How can current life be adjusted to earlier hopes and expectations?

The film itself is coquettish and clumsily didactic. It is like the movies of the 1950s, once seen in drive-ins, in which sex education was a cover for providing pleasure for lusting adolescents. In this post-AIDS film, the relationship between the screen narrative and the audience is achieved by making the leading actors into quasi-teachers, taking them out of the story so that they can confer with the viewer. And the lessons they teach are post-AIDS as well: You may seek the excitement of the early 1980s, in which "sex was still a good way to meet new people," but the sexual revolution is "something in the past." The two leading women, in their late twenties, journey to a health spa in southern California, where they seek at first the casual sexual relationships of their remembered (or anticipated) past. Humor allows the film to touch sensitive subjects. In the hotel room on their arrival is a bouquet of condoms in a ribboned basket. But the conclusion of this film is the most relevant thing about the post-AIDS movie industry. The consequence of their efforts is, ultimately, conversion to a Doris Day fifties marriage, with a Christmas tree and large dog, split-level house, children, and a changed sense of dress and of self. Safe sex is rejected for the safer sex of the mutually monogamous, happy marriage. It is as if the architecture of a new model of the ideal life is being worked out, awkwardly, on a thousand screens.

Casual Sex? is a fluff of a movie, but a telling one. The consciousness of the impact of AIDS is too explicit, too formally apparent—that is not the way we like our entertainment and education mixed. More subtle, but still specifically evocative, is the scene in *Broadcast News* in which the heroine surreptitiously places a condom in her purse on the way to a tryst with the handsome television anchorperson she loves. *Broadcast News* is a film more of the present, and while there are large numbers of exceptions, to be sure, the theme that casual sex is the norm, or even that it is generally acceptable, seems to be declining. For a modern-day James Bond, the numbers of objects of adoration have declined into the low single digits.

The 1988 Mike Nichols film *Working Girl* is a fable of the AIDS era. Confounding feminism and femininity, the film retains many past themes of sexual involvement, but with a softness and charm, a sincerity and regard for constancy and marriage that was less pronounced a decade ago. The movie is about a tough and attractive woman, an investment banker of the new breed, who is unknowingly engaged in a struggle with her more feeling, more feminine secretary both for a man and for her business position. Early in the film, singles bars and random affairs are depicted as somewhat sleazy. Both the secretary's lower-middle-class friends and the elite acquaintances of her new life are all aiming, in one way or another, toward marriage. "Being single is dangerous" is one of the first lines of the film. There are no one-night stands with strangers. No explicit sign of the condom need appear; the AIDS consciousness is present nonetheless.

A Language All Their Own

Music is the special language of the young, to the young. It has declared the independence of more than one generation. Rock music united young people from coast to coast, giving them a set of heroes and an intensely personal communications link— in essence, their own medium. It has been the foundation not only of its own empire but of empires of fashion and style. Rock music has affirmed ideas of freedom in the United States and subverted political systems inconsistent with freedom beyond American borders. The music industry, even more than the motion picture industry, has shaped the attitudes of the young toward sexual liberation since the 1960s.

A private and effective voice for cultural revolution, the rock music industry in the United States has enjoyed a strong and unencumbered adolescence. But in the face of a public health imperative that Americans, especially the young, change their conduct, the music industry is being asked to come of age. The maturity it is able to demonstrate as it weighs its various reponsibilities to its youthful audience will be of utmost interest to observers both in and out of government.

Whatever the message of any individual segment of rock music, the message of the genre as a whole has been to underscore a notion, perhaps ersatz, of autonomy, choice, and independence. The impact of rock music on the conduct of the young is thought to be extraordinary, though that conclusion is as much a product of intuition as of documentation. Still, for the teenage population that is the primary focus of AIDS-related education, rock music and its accoutrements are central to their image of themselves. The impact is made even stronger by the fact that youth themselves often create the music and lyrics. The special poetic codes of rock lyrics make them virtually and purposely inaccessible to all but their intended audience. This inherent privacy of the medium contributes to the confusion over intent and impact.

In the last decade, even prior to the AIDS crisis, strong efforts to curb the industry were made by an odd combination of the religious right, a group of concerned mothers called the Parents Music Resource Center, and occasionally feminists concerned with the exploitation of women. Their actions included demanding a rating system for rock music, encouraging disclosure of the lyrics, and trying to influence the choice of music played over the air by disc jockeys. In 1985, at Congressional hearings reminiscent of Powell's inquiries into the content of textbooks, Frank Zappa and John Denver took issue with the fundamental premises of those seeking to draw conclusions from ambivalent though admittedly raucous texts. Public health concerns relating to AIDS were still far in the future, and all sides were more cautious then about the desirability of direct government intervention than might now be the case.

In the eyes of many observers, the mere existence of these hearings calling for more collective responsibility in the music industry raised important First Amendment questions. The heavy burden in a free society, they maintained, was on those who were attacking rock based on their personal interpretation of the meaning of the songs of Prince, Twisted Sister, AC/DC, and others. Many people expressed discomfort with the idea that government should draw lines between the permissible and the impermissible in this context.

Distrust of the new music of each generation and of its impact on morals is a great American tradition. But in a public health crisis, the dynamic is far different. If there is a sustained, mass concern about modifying the behavior of the young for the purpose of protecting the public's health, then the arguments will take a wholly different form. Debating moral goals and determining whether a set of oblique messages is inconsistent with standards that cannot be agreed upon becomes beside the point. Unlike the hearings on the "meaning" of the lyrics of Prince, where the focus was on evidence of isolated suicides, theoretical impacts on psyches, or attenuated burdens of proof, the discussion in the AIDS era will center on the large-scale conflict between rock music's celebration of sexual activity and public health efforts to control the spread of infection. This invocation of public health is likely to have a far more compelling and unifying impact than did appeals to moral codes that are the subject of difference and debate.

Just as with motion pictures, the structure of the music industry is important to an understanding of how the content of music may change in light of the AIDS crisis. Music is perhaps the most democratic of the media. It is cheaply and universally available, and, in the form of the audio cassette, is easily duplicated and traded from hand to hand. The Walkman, with its ability to provide a private tent of communication between the listener and the musician, is perhaps the ultimate symbol of modern music's celebration of individual autonomy.

All this has given music a special force in the lives of the young and also has made it a more difficult area for control or influence by government. Even the Federal Communications Commission, which has sought to dampen appeals to prurience, has had enormous difficulty limiting language and innuendo on radio. To be sure, the regulated airwaves of radio are the major outlet for music. But federal hostility to regulation, competition from other unregulated technologies, and competitiveness within the industry make regulation virtually ineffective.

As concern about an AIDS epidemic heightens, the music world seems to be taking self-regulatory actions on its own. Jon Pareles in a *New York Times* article has demonstrated the change in song lyrics. "After decades in which opportunities to cut loose multiplied and consequences seemed to dwindle," he wrote, "pleasure has become suspect, even dangerous . . . Rock and pop songs, cultural artifacts that help define pleasure while they deliver it, are in a new bind: are they fantasies, chronicles of current mores, how-to's or teases?" Pareles saw an end to songs like Donna Summer's "Love to Love You Baby," in which "a beat, a melodic hook and moans galore suggested a world in which the party would go on forever with a sexuality that was tireless and polymorphous and all-embracing."[2].

Now, Janet Jackson urges, "Let's wait awhile, before we go too far"; Gwen Guthrie sings, "Love is no longer free / The price is high / I don't want no AIDS or herpes . . . I'm too young to die." New themes express a sense of shame for conduct that is socially unwise; they favor marriage and monogamy and affection without physical intimacy. The BBC, caught up in its sense of responsibility, banned George Michael's "I Want Your Sex" because of lyrics that stated, "Sex is natural—sex is good / Not everybody does it / But everybody should." On MTV, Michael's music video was reinstated only when the image for the song made monogamy a clearer context for the lyrics.

Prior to the AIDS crisis, the regulatory actions stimulated by rock music amounted to not much more than middle-aged head-wagging. And even then, the issue was not always sexual morality per se. In his essay on music in *The Closing of the American Mind*, Allan Bloom's concern is not with the moral effects of rock music but with its effect on education. His view is that the intense and early exposure of the young to rock harms the imagination and ultimately "makes it very difficult for [students] to have a passionate relationship to the art and thought that are the substance of liberal education."[3] But with AIDS, sexual activity itself is suddenly very much the issue with rock music. Is the extraordinary impact of music on the young hostile to a public health message that the state needs effectively to communicate? If the industry does not act responsibly, on its own initiative, and if the crisis worsens, the forces of censorship and control will turn to government once again.

Primetime Tutor

More than any other medium, television is the instrument that records the story mainstream America tells about itself and the life its members imagine themselves to lead. In an odd way, TV is the legacy of the official painting and sculpture of earlier times. We no longer commission statues of men on horseback for our parks, but we do have morality plays on television that establish a set of ethical rules for the decent conduct of our ordinary lives.

The traditional motivations of television executives have been twofold: to retain their ever-more-valuable television licenses, and to secure the confidence of advertisers, who are generally nervous about programming that diverges at all from middle-America's standards of morality.

The hand of the government in the television licensing process has been heavier than we often admit. Although censorship is explicitly forbidden, even the potential for review has contributed mightily to the restraint shown by producers for primetime programming. As an example, a little more than a decade ago the chairman of the Federal Communications Commission, responding to pressure from Congress and from groups around the country opposing excessive violence on television, held meetings with the heads of each of the three major networks to reduce what was thought to be the scourge of this programming for American youth. He obtained agreement from them to voluntarily establish a "family viewing time" in which industry-generated standards would be imposed to reduce the level of violence and bring the images shown on television up to some mediated ideal. Antitrust litigation eventually stopped this FCC-supervised effort of the networks, but the message had been clearly delivered and received.[4]

The FCC's standard for prohibiting programming on broadcast television and radio is "indecency" as well as obscenity.[5] The specific meaning of indecency is unclear, but broadcasters know that indecency may be reached well in advance of obscenity. And although broadcasters have been fighting for full First Amendment protection, they understand that pushing the indecency line is not the best way to gain Congressional support for their position.

When Congress debated how cable television should be regulated in the mid-1980s, one of the most important obstacles to consensus was the standard to be used to regulate cable television programming. One solution of Congress was to require cable operators to provide subscribers, on request, with a locking device that would give parents control over what channel was being watched.[6] The idea, perhaps too optimistic, was that programming could be more adventuresome, but that children would be protected.

Like members of Congress, but for different reasons, advertisers are also reluctant to risk offending the standards of decency of the vast primetime audience. The sitcom's seemingly innocuous conventions about family and sexuality, according to some industry analysts, are popular with advertisers because they attract large and passive audiences, sitting ducks for the much shorter, much more sexually charged hard-sell commercials. Even violence and car chases, for reasons that are deep within us, seem to reach and hold the attention of the many while offending only a few, and these shows too reappear season after season, decade after decade.

Partly because of the licensing process, partly because of the mass audience that they must deliver to the advertisers, television broadcasters do not take the chances that motion picture studios do. As a consequence, the impact of AIDS on television will be different from its impact on motion pictures or the music industry. Television programming has not been an engine for the assertion of individual freedom, as celebrated by sexual autonomy. Rather than feeling the need to reform its message away from this theme, television will feel the effect of AIDS in its odd function as a teaching medium. Though we think of television as largely escapist, it is, as a visual realization of the society the mainstream desires, blatantly instructionist. Thus it is not surprising that, from the miniseries to the situation comedy to the documentary, television programming is being used to get the message of AIDS to mainstream America. Even the evening news is an electronic pulpit, ever ready to deliver the sermons and speeches that emanate from Congress and other official spokespersons. The news has become a tool with which public health officials instruct people in how to think and how to behave during the AIDS crisis.

On television news, AIDS had at first been virtually ignored, largely, many thought, because of the character of the epidemic's victims. But after Rock Hudson's death, the existence of AIDS was daily hammered into the nation's consciousness, and the danger existed that coverage would more likely whip up scorn for the gay community rather than enhance understanding and aid public health initiatives. Coverage was less about sexuality and behavior than it was, in a sense, about the discovery by television of a frightful new battle zone. Deft use of language and symbols became of the greatest importance. Some responsible journalists sought to ensure that alarm did not translate into hatred for the gay subculture. Part of the task was to understand and transcend the general contempt of homosexuality that preceded AIDS and would be the referent for most viewers as they absorbed vast amounts of information in the period after 1982. Yet ironically, as Randy Shilts later reported, when NBC News was planning coverage of the 1984 Democratic Convention in San Francisco, it tried to make sure that gays would not be involved in the catering for its staff.[7]

Always present, though often beneath the surface, was concern that coverage of the epidemic could have its own impact on behavior. Sensitive efforts to further public health needs through careful education could drown in a climate of fear. To the extent that sound strategies depended on the coming forward of those infected or at risk, too terrifying a story of AIDS would hinder progress. And not only was it a question of discrimination and prejudice. News coverage could impugn the integrity of the blood supply, because of fear of infected donors; reports could cause undue hysteria among parents where children with AIDS were attending schools. Fear of using forbidden words was coupled, in the minds of network executives, with the fear of encouraging—or being seen to encourage—homosexuality. When NBC showed a drama about a young man in New York who contracts AIDS, the network censor cut elements of the script that could be seen as an endorsement of homosexuality. The hero's grandmother, for example, could not tell her grandson, "I think your boyfriend is nice." At the end of the drama, after young Michael dies, there is a closing shot of a family album, all united, but Michael's friend is excluded.

So vital is the question of how people are depicted in AIDS-related dramas that there are now negotiations between producers and representatives of gay organizations. In 1988, Lorimar showed an episode of the television program *Midnight Caller* about a bisexual man in San Francisco who was knowingly spreading the AIDS virus through sexual promiscuity. In the original script, the talk-radio personality who is the star of the program tracks down the villain, and the episode was to end in his violent death. After tense discussions with gay civil rights groups, Lorimar radically altered the program, softening the ending and representing the sense of responsibility and compassion that has been characteristic of the gay response to AIDS. Yet even after these changes in the script, the finished program was condemned by AIDS leaders: by portraying an individual with AIDS as a killer out to infect others, television was, they said, exhibiting the callousness and ignorance that ignites and perpetuates discrimination and violence.

The clumsy difficulty of serving as a mirror of the society and a moral tutor at a time of change is illustrated by the programming of CBS one summer evening in 1987. To much fanfare, the network showed *An Enemy among Us,* a program about a young middle-class boy who tested AIDS-positive as a result of receiving a blood transfusion several years before. It was state-of-the-art AIDS instruction, with Gladys Knight delivering a lecture to a classroom of students about the need to postpone sexual relations. "The free-wheeling days of the 60s and 70s are over," she said. This brave attempt to chasten America's youth was followed by the fifth annual Miss Teen America Contest, featuring, as role models, the cheerleaders of the Dallas Cowboys, along with fifty-one contestants singing a sultry version of "I Wonder Who's Hot Tonight." The ironies did not end there, however. Among the advertisements was a commercial for an eye-coloring brush, called a Stick Wand, whose shape, according to accepted advertising doctrine, is designed to inspire happy associations with the male sex organ.

But the Stick Wand is part of advertising, not programming. When we examine commercials, we find quite a different relationship between the curriculum of the 1970s and 80s and the public health needs of the AIDS era.

Haiku of Desire

Advertising in general, and television commercials in particular, are more powerful than most other creative efforts at driving home the triple whammy of individualism, choice, and sexual freedom. This medium therefore presents a forbidding obstacle to those who would alter our images of proper sexual behavior during the AIDS crisis. Here is ideology put in the service of consumerism, and it is a forceful combination. Advertising is firmly grounded in the principle of choice, in the commitment to convincing each consumer that he or she is a free person, free to choose, and free to exercise that choice through the selection of consumer goods. And it was long ago discovered that when the desire to consume is joined with the desire to consummate, the compulsion to buy is intensified.

Marshall McLuhan early argued that consumerism and sexuality are closely linked. Cars, perfume containers, deodorant sticks, all have been configured as sexual objects to enhance sales. Lucy Komisar wrote in the early 1970s about the "obvious attempt to promote sexual fantasies with soap advertising." She cited what seemed to be an effort "to project a virtual love affair between housewife and soap-suds." Ultra Brite toothpaste was designed to "give your mouth sex appeal." Colgate mouthwash is "the mouthwash for lovers." And, as Komisar reported almost twenty years ago, "An ad for bath oil shows a man embracing a woman while the copy blazes away: 'Sardo. When you live with a man.' "[9]

The commercials of the 1950s and 1960s have been attacked by feminists, not necessarily for showing the sexuality of housewives but for showing women generally with a husband and always in need of authority. Enter the commercials of the 1970s, the era of the liberated female consumer. This woman has "come a long way, Baby" as a role model; she buys a great many things to enhance her sexuality, and she enhances it, in large part, to demonstrate her independence, her freedom, and her range of choice. The stories of the 1980s are different still from those of the 1970s, in that they imply immediate sexual payoffs. The pioneers of the 1980s—Calvin Klein, Guess? Chanel—have created an art form out of this new image of the American woman and her potential. There is a harsh mystery and taut sensuality to the new woman, a seeming fulfillment of independence (though one that is bitterly attacked by some feminists because the independence itself is founded on a need for alluring sexuality). In Riunite wine advertisements, the process of swallowing raspberries has set a new standard in sexual suggestiveness.

If motion pictures are the narrative of sexual relations in the 1980s, commercials have been their haiku. From jeans to chewing gum, the extraordinarily compact and highly produced stories in commercials are exquisitely designed to fuel autonomy, an intense sense of self, and the idea of the ever more fabulous conquest, and to implicitly criticize lives that are drab, bland, and therefore not in need of the embellishments that symbolize pursuit. Buying a product is portrayed as a prerequisite to fulfilling sexual dreams, or at least facilitating their fulfillment. Indeed, sometimes the product sold *is* the dream, or at least the dream and the product are indistinguishable. And as the focus of marketing has changed to the young and well-heeled, away from the paradigmatic Midwestern family, the nature of the dreams that are the foundation of commercial fulfillment have changed. The dream of a satisfied, though stereotype-drenched, family life has more and more given way to dreams of a freer, more casual life, less bound by rules, by monogamy or sexual loyalty, less bound, in sum, by other people, more bound up in the concept of self.

So this is the situation of that most polished and public of creative forms at the threshold of the AIDS crisis. If we are concerned about television as one of the shapers of our identities, we must be even more concerned with the meaning of commercials. The producers of advertising have been masters of the use of television to imprint an idealized society on our minds. They have proclaimed a society to exist in which the action of consuming goods has been transformed into a moral imperative, in which happiness in love is linked with fulfillment in consumption. They are the counterparts to the forceful molders of culture in government-controlled central economies. Advertising has been the pre-eminent proof of the power of the media to shape habits, to change culture, to affect patterns of life. Indeed, the idea of the free, unencumbered individual, the maker of decisions, is as critical for the foundation of advertising as he or she is for the foundation of democratic theory.

The advertising industry has not been impervious to the AIDS crisis. Television advertisements for Paco Rabanne, a French men's perfume, illustrate how AIDS consciousness is already affecting commercial messages. In the 1982 television campaign, a man lies in bed, satisfied, covered with sheets of silk. A phone rings: "Hello," the man answers. "You snore," a woman says. "And you steal the covers," he retorts. In the 1988 advertisement, a new Paco Rabanne man blows a kiss to the air, descends a winding stairway, walks down cobblestone streets and across a bridge, enraptured in a fantasy about the previous evening. The creator of the new commercial attributes the difference to AIDS: "Fantasy and romance are in; explicit sex isn't."[10]

Television finds ways of adjusting sexuality to the constraints of AIDS. Love and sexuality have found a new place of notoriety within marriage. An advertisement for Hyatt Hotels, soft-core, bodies moving in silken sheets, is at great pains to show the woman of the pair with a wedding band on her finger. Epilady, a maker of depilatories, arouses zeal for its product by depicting a very long, very inviting leg, but concludes with a clearly ring-bearing hand stroking its smoothness. Oldsmobile, as in days of old, suggests the power of a car to assure happiness in love, but increasingly, through the symbol of the ring, marriage is an implicit part of the visual text. Here, advertising is reinforcing trends elsewhere. *Cosmopolitan* magazine features a story on "taking the monotony out of monogamy," and advice-column letters in *Penthouse* are increasingly about sexuality within marriage, as opposed to without.

On the other hand, inconsistent with the imperatives of AIDS is the tendency of the networks, because of the force of competition, to become more hospitable to explicit sexuality in the exercise of their acceptance or "clearance" standards. Faced with a shrinking audience, because of the competition from cable and other new video forms, network executives strive harder to keep advertising revenues strong. If one network relaxes its practices about sexual explicitness in advertising, then the other networks find it hard to resist the pressing of established boundaries by those who advertise with them.

Government regulation of advertising, even of television commercials, has been virtually nonexistent as they relate to the new sexuality, and regulation imposed from within the industry has been trivial. Even that low level of self-regulation steadily diminished as a result of a bizarre action by the U.S. Department of Justice in the mid-1980s. Until then, the National Association of Broadcasters had followed a self-imposed program of standards in advertising. But the Department of Justice claimed these standards violated antitrust laws because they were an agreement among competitors to limit competition.

Controversy over the content of broadcast television commercials and the message they send to the society emerged in the early 1970s over advertising for cigarettes. Many argued that these commercials had two messages: one for the specific brand of cigarette, and another, implicit, that advocated the practice of smoking itself. This second message, it was argued, raised a controversial issue of public importance and, under the then-existing fairness doctrine, stations had a duty to broadcast commercial messages that proclaimed another view—that smoking was dangerous. For a variety of reasons, one of which was the power of the antismoking ads, the cigarette companies acquiesced in federal legislation that banned cigarette advertising in the regulated media. It was a way of keeping the antismoking ads off the television screen.

As a result of the FCC's penchant for deregulation, there is little of the fairness doctrine alive today. Consequently, no forum exists in which to argue that many ads subliminally present only one side in a current controversial debate of public importance, namely, what personal sexual practices should be encouraged in the face of the AIDS epidemic. But stations themselves have already demonstrated their willingness to carry public service advertisements that advocate changed behavior. It remains to be seen how fervently these stations will refuse to broadcast commercials that promote sexual practices discouraged by public health officials. More to the point, one may ask whether their public service programming—their documentaries and news accounts—adequately countervail the impact of product advertising.

One would have thought that a major impact of the AIDS crisis on the advertising industry, and on television commercials in particular, would be a dramatic change in the permissibility of promoting condoms. Prior to AIDS, the NAB Code prohibited television commercials for condoms or any other prophylactic product. The Surgeon General and the Centers for Disease Control are advocates for far more extensive use of condoms for safer sex. It ought to be considered a sign of responsibility to show condom ads, and the advertising industry has been enormously creative about ways to present the use of condoms so as to enhance the public health process without implicitly encouraging sexual conduct among the young. Yet as the AIDS epidemic entered its second decade, no network and few local stations showed condom ads, with the exception of random public service announcements.

But condom advertising alone should not be the litmus test for whether or not the industry is acting with foresight and care. The strong fables about autonomy and sexuality that the industry creates for society have contributed greatly to the American identity, and ultimately it is this very identity that is at stake as concerns about public health mount.

Scared Sexless

Every day, in newspapers, in television programs, in political speeches, the struggle to properly shape the image of AIDS and reshape our sense of personhood is newly engaged. Each story, each anecdote, each event is a cue as to whether to become more fearful or more compassionate, more confident or more concerned about the capacity of government and medicine to deal with this crisis. Each story has within it, consciously or not, a bundle of messages about the expertise of government and medicine, about how individuals should behave, what is expected of them, what constitutes responsibility.

At the end of 1987, NBC broadcast an hour-long program primarily directed at bringing teenagers and singles up to date on the implications of AIDS for their behavior. The program, *Scared Sexless*, displayed the conflicts and tensions in American society that influence how the AIDS crisis is depicted and how the significance of the crisis is absorbed and translated into everyday life.

There was Connie Chung, consummate anchorperson and interlocutor, solitary on the screen, authoritatively determined to guide us through the uncertainties of AIDS. She exemplified the general desire in the community for answers. This was television at its most successful and reassuring, with anchor as surrogate, the voice of every person, given the opportunity and endowed with the resources to ask questions and communicate the answers. The impression inherent in a network news and documentary presentation is one of objectivity and comprehensiveness. The audience is ostensibly being presented with an understanding and some resolution of a complex and intensely troubling subject. A network television program is often a looking-glass of sorts: Almost by definition, it must hallow and incorporate the collection of ideas and background that the American public brings to its crises. Like all television programs, *Scared Sexless* was a cultural artifact, a rosetta stone whose message, as well as what it omits from that message, tells us a good deal about the society in which it was produced.

Scared Sexless was one of the most-watched documentaries of the year, indicating the heightened consciousness and apprehension concerning AIDS and the hunger for information and reassurance. Because this was a significant program, dealing with a subject of great sensitivity, there were few accidents in its production. It was a purposeful documentary that embodied and reflected many of the current tensions in American culture while trying to make a factual presentation of AIDS issues.

Standing alone on a darkened set among a group of empty brass bedsteads, Connie Chung opened the program by stating that a significant percentage of people infected with AIDS are not from the high-risk groups thought to dominate the ranks of AIDS victims, and that in Africa most of the spread of AIDS has been through heterosexual intercourse. Immediately, the program was taking a stance in the struggle over how AIDS should be depicted—AIDS, she was asserting, is a generalized threat, a dilemma that affects the community at large. By underscoring AIDS as being of increasing danger to heterosexuals, the aim of the program was to jolt awake people who consider themselves in line with the sexual norms of society and therefore protected from the ravages of AIDS. This was a program addressed to, and about, mainstream, heterosexual Americans. It sought to strike the nerves of people who cheat on their spouses, of singles leading hit-or-miss sex lives, of teenage sweethearts attending the school prom.

In one part of the program there appeared, almost as a paradigm, a sweet boy and girl, high school seniors, who regularly sleep together with the knowledge of their parents. Connie Chung interviewed the mothers, who spoke of the cautions taken to ensure that the sexual relations of the young couple are not endangering their health. Though a random example of behavior, this case history takes on the stature of a synedochal symbol. This particular teenage couple's adjustments to life in modern society, and the liberal supervision by parents who symbolize the community at large, are supposed to stand for the general relationship all Americans should endeavor to maintain. The message was clear: We must adjust, but we can remain essentially the same.

The lesson emanating from government was similarly reassuring: There is no reason to panic; your society is doing everything it can to find a vaccine for AIDS; our researchers are the world's best; they are motivated, they have the resources; there will probably be a solution; in the meantime, AIDS means changing your personal conduct. But these changes, according to the program, will not damage the existing fabric of American life. Just a little condom will do the trick.

As the AIDS crisis has intensified, programs like *Scared Sexless* have repeatedly faced the question of whether to depict the epidemic as a moral issue or a public health issue. The sharp division and insecurity in the country over the nature of morality, religious teaching, and their connection to sexuality was resolved by the NBC program, that December night, by not calling upon any religious figures or ethicists to indicate their perspectives on ways to alter conduct. The view that public health messages should stress abstinence was relegated to a lone White House official, a bureaucrat lacking in persuasiveness. AIDS, for NBC, was strictly a public health matter, not a moral matter. The solution was primarily a technical one.

Not surprisingly, ironies abounded as the network struggled with the permissible range of representations, with the images that could be shown, the words that could be used. A lengthy segment of *Scared Sexless* dealt with condoms, showing how they are manufactured, how they are tested, how they can fail. Here was a straightforward message about preventive measures—"safer sex," in the jargon of the moment. Yet the local stations that carried this network program did not, as a matter of policy, broadcast advertisements for condoms. Moreover, in a kind of witless misadventure that is so revealing, one of the commercials during the program—an advance promotion for *An Officer and A Gentleman*—showed Debra Winger passionately making love with Richard Gere. The mix of images presented by the documentary was only a visual escape from the real dilemma our society must face. The program appeared neutral, but it was not. Buried in the coolly edited presentation was a deeply felt conflict in the society between our fear and our fantasies.

Scared Sexless was interesting, too, because of the way it reflected changes in gender roles in the society. NBC was particularly careful about the images of men and women that it chose. In emphasizing safer sex as the most important element of public health education, the documentary implicitly rejected the macho image of the postadolescent male who measures his worth by the number of his female conquests. It also implicitly rejected the image of young women as passive, not demanding of consideration from their boyfriends, as victims both of social pressures and personal domination. Yet in a segment that featured frank discussions with young men—with a male airline steward interviewed with a group of flight attendants, male and female, and with star football player Marcus Allen—the program exposed the flaw in making these assumptions about male–female relationships. There was Allen, in his trophy-lined study, model of achievement and male apotheosis, being asked if he still celebrated life as a successful object of physical adoration, as a stud on the road. His answer was no, but it was not all that convincing. The embarrassed look, the snicker, acknowledged a fast-paced life, or at least the hope for one, in which freedom from sexual constraints is taken for granted. The nervous young steward, when asked about his sexual practices, defensively asserted—despite the contradictory opinions of his female friends—that he did not always insist on condoms, that they interfered with his sexual pleasure and his idea of himself. Two men, then, very different, both commenting on their relationship to the great tradition of maleness in our society and how uncomfortable they were as that tradition was coming under assault.

It was not by accident that the program's principal interlocutor—the guide—was a woman, and one, like Ms. Chung, whose persona is strong and controlled, yet feminine, a woman who has succeeded by being somewhat different, or perhaps in spite of being somewhat different. Like Ms. Chung, the other women in the program were the people who were most in control of themselves and of change, who were confident, cool, learning to be safe and to stay safe. The prototype of the young, single woman was a comedienne in New York who works hard, who uses her tough wit as a shield, whose life has been a history of coping. The stewardesses, models of male fantasy, also asserted that their styles of life have changed. And when the program turned to the young high school lovers, it was the mothers, not the fathers, who were in charge of determining that their sexual relations were not putting them at risk of disease.

By nuance and inference the program sought, as well, to place distance between those who are responding "properly" and those who were clinging to pre-AIDS cultural norms. Singles bars were depicted as places of loneliness, not as trendy cultural innovations. A bartender mused about the understandable dropoff in business. At the counter, people were seen dimly, through a haze of smoke and lights, drinking, virtually abandoned.

Here then is the complex situation with respect to the media as our society undertakes the task of defining risk and educating itself anew as to proper conduct. The culture has become suffused, through the media, with an appreciation of freedom of choice and autonomy of the individual, both associated, very strongly, with sexual achievement and sexual choice. The motor of the consumer society for two decades has been adjusted to this set of images. Some products are directly dependent on this set of messages, and many products have been closely identified with them.

The AIDS crisis is bringing pressure to alter this image of sexuality in American life. In New York and Los Angeles, news of glittering charity benefits, attended by movie stars, rock musicians, and industry executives, fill the society pages as money is raised for AIDS services, research, and treatment. The question is how high these impulses to respond in times of national emergency otherwise rank in the minds of often cynical business leaders. Entertainment executives have themselves personally seen the ravages of AIDS and suffered the loss of valued talent; they cannot help but see, in the need to control the disease, the irony of their own glorification of behavior that is potentially destructive. They also will not fail to notice that audiences themselves are building new ways of interpreting sexual imagery. Scenes of passion that once triggered feelings of desire now trigger thoughts of contagion in the minds of many moviegoers. Today, casual sex, like cigarette smoking, delivers at best a mixed message.

Finally, corporate America also knows that if the crisis intensifies, pressure from government could become enormous. Groups that historically have sought to constrain the media will have powerful allies and a stronger argument for government intervention. What they lacked before—some legitimate reason why government should choose their standard over that of others—is provided by the public health need.

So change may be occurring, change in the stories that film and television tell, that music plays. Even advertising is slowly shifting, however difficult and expensive it is to alter the identification and sense of a product. "Hollywood is talking about getting around to recognizing that the backseat of the limousine, first time out, can lead to the grave," A. M. Rosenthal wrote, starkly, in 1987. "But aside from one or two pictures, it still is all to come later."[11]

The pace of change will be determined by how important it is to government that a public health message be effectively communicated. The government's messages cannot be successful if they must do battle with the competing voices of commerce and the arts. Self-change is preferable to censorship. But the government's role in defining the relationship between public health and private lives may increase. If it does, the consequence will be a change in the way we think about law, speech, and culture.[12]

two

The Voice of Government
in the Marketplace of Ideas

As the federal government mobilizes its public education effort
to combat the further spread of the AIDS virus, the obvious
First Amendment issues are not the most likely ones to present
problems. Should the government eventually try to regulate the
scripts of motion pictures or tell bookstores what publications
they can and cannot distribute, that would be censorship, and
our society has a strong tradition of legal scholarship against
which these actions could be analyzed. The government's response to AIDS is not likely to take so clear and dictatorial a
style, at least not right away, given the growing sensitivity of
the media to public health needs and the voluntary actions they
have taken thus far. More likely than censorship—and in fact
already under way—is a direct effort by the government to affect
the way the public thinks about AIDS by delivering powerful
messages of its own, in its own voice. The meaning of the First
Amendment to the Constitution—that "Congress shall make
no law . . . abridging the freedom of speech, or of the press"—
is far less clear in this area of government speech.

   The First Amendment is a legal text, and as such it is open
to many interpretations. But the First Amendment is also a
symbol, and how it is understood as a symbol at any given time
determines to a large extent how it will be interpreted by judges.
To understand more concretely how a political symbol's meaning can change drastically over time, we need look no further
than New York Harbor. When the Statue of Liberty was inau-

gurated there in 1886, its symbolic meaning had little, if anything, to do with the stream of immigrants to the United States. The complete name of this huge monument with its beacon raised was Liberty Enlightening the World, and its symbolic meaning in those early years centered on exporting our political system, not importing immigrants. By 1986, at the time of the statue's centennial, the meaning of the great figure had been almost completely transformed. Liberty had become a symbol of the United States as receiver, as melting pot, as the great democratic experiment. The statue's new meaning was formally expressed in the words of the poet Emma Lazarus, "Give me your tired, your poor, your huddled masses yearning to breathe free . . ." which in 1883 had been engraved on Liberty's base.[1] Towering above Ellis Island, the chief immigration station of the country from 1892 to 1943, the Statue of Liberty had come to symbolize the promise of a new life in a free land.

The First Amendment is not a physical metaphor like the Statue of Liberty, but it too is an icon of our society. And, like the meaning of other complex symbols, the way the First Amendment is perceived by the community changes over time, owing to countless reverberations and references, to conscious and unconscious repetitions and descriptions of it. Moreover, there is probably a strong connection between the public's perception of what the First Amendment means and the way it is interpreted by a judge in a particular case. Indeed, the shifting of the symbolic sense of the First Amendment over time may be responsible for substantial changes in its legal interpretation.

If this is the way judicial interpretation comes about, then the AIDS crisis is likely to be a powerful influence on the way our legal system views free speech in the future. AIDS is the kind of strong background event that can shape the psyche, that can establish a hidden framework for thinking about images and their meaning. It is the kind of event that tends to redefine the role of government in the public mind. In the face of a growing need for public education powerful enough to change personal behavior in so vital an area as sexual relations, members of the community and judges on the bench may both discover that the symbolic meaning we have attached to the First Amendment for the past fifty years is inadequate.

At the center of this fifty-year-old tradition is the concept of the "marketplace of ideas." It assumes that everyone's ideas, no matter how controversial, should be given free expression, unrestrained by government intervention; that if individuals are encouraged to think and speak freely, and to attempt to sway public opinion from their soapboxes, eventually truth will win out. As one scholar of the marketplace view has summarized it, "We allow people to speak so others can vote. Speech allows people to vote intelligently and freely, aware of all the options and in possession of all the relevant information."[2] But the pursuit of truth is not limited to political truth. As the tradition of the marketplace of ideas has emerged, political speech, literary and artistic speech, and commercial speech are all protected, partly because there are no useful ways to distinguish among them. The marketplace of ideas gives the nod to the winner both in ideology, in cultural styles, and in advocacy of various modes of consumption.

The AIDS crisis has jolted our confidence in this view of free speech, at least insofar as, unfettered, it has produced cultural ideas and habits that are a risk to the public's health. The crisis has forced us to look at the dominant messages that free expression has produced and to demand at a minimum that government more actively enter the marketplace and itself speak forcefully so as to counter them.

Public efforts to change behavior are the quintessential hallmark of the strategy to slow the spread of AIDS. When mandatory testing is suggested as a strategy, it is denounced as counterproductive, because it would force possible carriers of the AIDS virus underground. When closing or regulation of bathhouses was first advocated in San Francisco and New York, again, the telling argument was that, above all, the environment for education, for persuasion to alter behavior, was the better mode. We have staked our all on a concerted attempt to change attitudes through education. And here, education is nothing more than a euphemism for government efforts directly or indirectly to urge styles of life and styles of aspiration sometimes radically different from what went before.

How can this vital task be accomplished if other signals in our society compete in a destructive manner with those of government? Granted, each day commercial television networks, newspapers, and other media are finding ways to enrich public understanding of AIDS and improve the public debate on AIDS-related questions. But the need for a disciplined set of communications may be more than the marketplace of ideas, unaided and undirected, can manage. The pace of change may be too slow, and in the interim people may be confused by the conflicting signals they receive from the media. The notion is that a strong enough government voice, instructing the fearful populace as to desirable behavior, may offset the confusion arising from the conflicting messages in the rest of the culture.

Minding the Children

In trying to understand the role that government speech may play in shaping public opinion in a calculated way, perhaps the easiest place to start is with children. If pressure continues to build for public health education to prevent the spread of AIDS, nowhere will that pressure be greater than with respect to the young. Children, rising into adolescence, are the most moldable. Their attitudes are most keenly affected by the customs, mores, and value systems that permeate the media. They are the primary consumers of music, movies, even television, and as consumers they are wonderfully, even charmingly, impressionable. It is understandable that the simple marketplace model, in which everyone is encouraged to say what he or she wants in order to sway behavior, is less acceptable in relation to the young. For that reason, government has long been called upon to formally educate them, rather than leave the molding of their ideas totally to the vicissitudes of personal experience.

In the AIDS crisis, school districts across the country have already begun programs of AIDS education, and the propriety of the various messages about health and sex being addressed to the young in this setting has been the subject of much discussion.

Because the young are so central to our thinking about the proper mix of speech in the community, more needs to be said about what images we have in mind of children and the family when we think about how speech is absorbed and how it affects conduct and attitudes. This is particularly true when we deal with the affirmative role of government as teacher in the AIDS crisis; the tie is close between the public health message and a kind of public morality that could be inferred from it.

The principal bulwark for the tradition of free speech—the emphasis on the responsibility of the individual—works as applied to children only if one assumes that it is the individuality of the *parents*, not the children, that is at stake. We want to protect the right of the family to mold the child, to establish the moral and cultural environment in which the child will be reared and the framework by which the child interprets the world. The autonomy protected is the autonomy of the family. Government influence should be limited, it has been felt, because the family, not Big Brother, should make decisions about how attitudes of children should be shaped.

But there are two Americas to consider when we think about the education of our children. One is the romantic and idealized America, the America of the father and the mother and two or three children, the America of the family farm, the America of the pleasant suburb or the city of immigrants struggling to prepare their offspring for a productive future in a free land. The other is the statistical America, a growing America, reflected in the work of sociologists and census takers, where so many children do not have parents in charge, where parents, for a complex of reasons, have abdicated the role of moral tutor or feel that their role has been usurped by influences beyond their control.

I see myself and my family as part of the first America. My wife and I have three children. We have tried diligently to provide an excellent education for them and to exemplify good moral precepts and impart good civic attitudes. Worrying about our children, what they read, who their friends are, what they intend to do with their future, how they take to schooling—all have taken up a substantial part of our psychic identities. It is a costly and time-consuming process. We could do better, but we have done all right.

But it would be horrid to commit the dangerous fallacy of establishing national policy on the basis that family life conforms to a norm in which parents alone perform and are capable of performing the role of establishing some set of values in their children. Some, like Margaret Mead, would argue that parents, in general, do not play this role and that in many societies it is performed by grandparents or extended families. Indeed, it is not our national policy to assume that education can be or is left to parents. Compulsory-education laws and the whole system of public education are a recognition of this fact.

The point is that the second America is strongly dominant. It is not a conclusion that I like to reach or one that should give anybody comfort. But it should be recognized so that a suitable local, state, and national policy can be fashioned. If our ideal of how values are transferred from generation to generation does not adequately reflect reality, it cannot prove a useful guide to shaping policy.

In our own not-too-distant past, extended family, along with religious institutions, helped parents define values and transfer them to children. Local government, largely through the public schools, also assumed part of the responsibility. But with time, church and extended family lost their force in our society, and moral education in the public schools slid out of fashion. Over the same period, the media, particularly the electronic media, began to permeate the culture and, one could argue, have gradually become our society's substitute teachers in the realm of values.

One gets a clue into the changing role of parents by looking at the books they generally read to their children. It may be a small observation, but the ratio of pictures to words in these books seems to have increased geometrically over the years. A greater proportion of children's books for the young are predominantly composed of illustrations. The heavy texts, those that required the reading of a chapter a night, seem to have vanished to the margin. Many reasons explain this change, including, of course, the rise of television. But one condition for highly textual children's books is the availability of literate readers to children and, for a variety of reasons, few of them (parents or extended family) may now exist or think that such reading is the highest value.

More relevant is that many modern children's books are almost wholly without large-scale morals. They are, almost without exception, devoid of nationalistic or patriotic messages. This is an enormous change. The emphasis now is increasingly on teaching children step-by-step skills or skills of human understanding and group relations, or imaginative flights of fancy. Think of the bestsellers among children's books. Richard Scarry teaches words and the association between words and pictures. Others teach whimsy and rhyme as a threshold to better reading. Many books are aimed at increasing a child's sense of wonder, fantasy, or understanding of other people or lines of work.

These are not like the children's books of a century or half century ago, the books of moral tales, like Aesop's fables, or great myths, like Pandora's box. They are not even like Robert McCloskey's celebrations of small-town America. Our children's books are successful at many things, but, with important exceptions, they seem to steadfastly stay away from value-rich messages. It is possible that authors avoid grand statements on the theory that today's parents think of them as overly interventionist, inconsistent with their more value-free approach to the bringing up of children. All these considerations and factors affect the marketplace of ideas for children and the range of children's choice among them.

Programs like *The Cosby Show* aside, the evolution of commercial television programming similarly reflects this drive toward the eschewing of values. Because the plethora of cable networks provides a veritable museum of black-and-white sitcoms of twenty and more years ago, it is easy to see how television itself has changed in the last thirty years. Here we are not dealing with the ancient and heavy bookish mythmaking of the Brothers Grimm but simply moralistic series such as *Lassie* or *The Ozzie and Harriet Show*. Maybe these shows are not being made today because there is more of a conflict over what values are the correct values, or perhaps there is conflict over whether values, as values, are something that should be vaunted at all. Perhaps it is thought that values—associated with a story line—do not command so large an audience as programs that are clear of values or are antivalue. Perhaps the advertisers' goal of greater and flashier consumerism has been increasingly inconsistent with simple moral tales.

If we look at books, television, and music in terms of degree of parental scrutiny and intervention in selection, we find that by and large parents select the books children see or the books that are read to them but are much less involved in selecting television programming. Last in the hierarchy of parental involvement is music, which has come to be the lingua franca among children, a private zone that parents usually do not invade. The accessibility of music, the low cost of acquiring or trading for it, the manner in which it is heard—all of these place music at a far lower level of parental intervention than books or television.

Of course not one of these modes is devoid of values. Perhaps ironically, music may be the medium most robust with values, though they may not always be the conventional ones. For those young people who think that we are living in a time of national hypocrisy, adherence to the appearance of traditional values in music lyrics, and in dress and behavior, may be the same as betraying their very essence. And conversely, adherence to seemingly rebellious lifestyles may cover a true respect for traditions or an oblique demand that values be concretely stated.

Values are hard to identify, hard to spot, especially if they are delicately included in the diet of our lives. We do not know what messages and morals children absorb from television programs and commercials, from motion pictures and comic books, or from the omnipresent music. To some adults, children's cartoons seem vapid or violent, the comic books filled with meaningless mythology, the music merely an assemblage of unintelligible concatenations. But children may be receiving a different message. It is interesting that, when given the choice, children will often choose material that is highly moralistic, highly value-laden, highly charged with issues of national political concern.

And of course programming or publications directed to the young are not the only media influences they encounter. Useful as it would be to segregate speech directed to children from speech in general, this is almost impossible to do. To be sure, at the margin, "adult bookstores" and peep shows, as well as X-rated movies, are prohibited from admitting children. But for television, radio, and advertising, messages that are generally available to adults are also available to children. The Federal Communications Commission, in addressing the problem of children's exposure to "offensive" words on television, concluded that there was hardly a time of day or night that was presumptively not in the zone of concern.[3] Though the FCC retreated somewhat from this position, we might still conclude that children are no longer ghettoized, for better or worse. Not only are they heard as well as seen, but they hear as well as see virtually everything. The inverse of this is that, because the young are being admitted to the society of adults sooner, we are all, in some way, at risk of being treated—by the media or by the government—as children.

Perhaps it is because we are insecure or unknowing about the cumulative lessons of these myriad thundering influences on the young that some people, in the face of the AIDS crisis, call for a simpler and clearer articulation by the government of a set of moral ideas. So far the call is not for censorship but for government to aggressively help mold how children think, particularly about sexual behavior. Dispute rages over what exactly the message should be and how it best should be communicated, but the demand for the government to help ensure that a different mix of messages reaches our children is clearly being felt.

This call for government intervention in the marketplace is, of course, far from new. The growth of the public school movement is testimony to how ingrained it is in the American tradition. Another, more recent, example is public television. Our system of noncommercial television is different from that of other countries, primarily because of First Amendment doubts about the propriety of a national, government-controlled communications vehicle. Those constitutional doubts are not minor, but the main point here is that public television has been used, and quite effectively, by the government to improve the nature and working of the marketplace of ideas as it directly affects children.

The use of public television for this purpose was a deliberate, strategic decision by the government, taken largely because of a sense that, without government intervention, the marketplace was resulting in inadequate substantive messages to its audience. Report after report, study after study, demonstrated that without any form of government coercion or intervention, the television programming served up to children would have, on the whole, little redeeming value. Government had tried, from time to time, to urge the networks and local stations to carry "good" children's programming. But there had not been great success, and First Amendment issues restrained government from forcing stations to meet national needs. A major reason for the formation and justification of a public television system was such children's programming of distinction as *Reading Rainbow*, *Sesame Street*, and *Mister Rogers*.

We have accomplished this in the United States in a very circuitous manner. Still, public television stands as one way of having the federal government intervene to improve the quality of the dialogue in the society, the quality of education. Here was a recognition that the marketplace of ideas, including television as well as schools, had not been, absent some government intervention, adequately providing educational and value-related products for our children. Only through enriching communications, through taking a positive step, was some corrective in the marketplace possible.

Now this way of looking at government's role in the area of speech is a potentially troubling one. Positive government intervention can be as worrisome as government abridgment of speech, at least if done without care. Government could crowd out other speakers if it were so inclined and so permitted. And the existence of an independent government voice could lead, even unintentionally, to establishing policies that would harm nongovernment competitors.

Appropriately, we in the United States have been sensitive to the question of the content of the government's message. In the case of public television, part of the genius of the American system has been that none of the programming is actually produced by a government agency or even agencies controlled by the government. And much of the financing for production is from private sources, so that dependence does not lead to its own infirmities. Most of these precautions grew out of the fear that a set of government messages on morality and public attitude would be stifling, wrong, and inconsistent with our tradition; they would yield a kind of secularized version of an established church.

Dangers have arisen and been thwarted in the past as government intervened to "help" children. In many localities in the nineteenth and twentieth centuries, after the formation of public schools, there were restrictions on alternate forms of schooling that a child could receive. In the 1920s, an Oregon law was passed requiring every child to attend public school. In striking it down, the U.S. Supreme Court said that "the child is not the mere creature of the state; those who nurture him and direct his destiny have the right, coupled with the high duty, to recognize and prepare him for additional obligations."[4] At the same time, however, Justice McReynolds acknowledged that the state can regulate schools, to assure that "teachers shall be of good moral character and patriotic disposition, that certain studies plainly essential to good citizenship must be taught, and that nothing be taught which is manifestly inimical to the public welfare."[5] In an earlier case, *Meyer v. Nebraska*, the Court struck down a statute that prohibited a child from going to a German-language school.[6] In the special case of the Amish, *Wisconsin v. Yoder*,[7] a 1972 Supreme Court decision upheld the right of a distinct religious minority to withold its children from schools after the eighth grade, despite local mandatory school-attendance laws. But even here, the Court recognized the extraordinary power of the state. It narrowly limited freedom from the power of the state to those parents who can assert that they are engaging in traditional religious upbringing and through that upbringing preparing their children for adult obligations in the society of which they will be a part. Thus we learn how tricky, how pervasive, any positive step by government into the lives of our children can be. When the state intervenes, institutions spring into being and then need to be protected—the empire of public education becomes its own vested interest.

One can hardly imagine that a proposed set of values cleared for promulgation by the government would encourage rebellious individuality. In the mildly successful Alan Alda film *Sweet Liberty*, one character playfully lists three prerequisites for a motion picture directed at a youthful audience: the action must show (1) disrespect for authority; (2) destruction of property, and (3) someone in the nude. Perhaps it is central to a budding sense of freedom and democracy among the young that they have a healthy mistrust for authority; and perhaps in a materialistic society the destruction of property by a few might even be a useful antidote to enshrining it. Whatever the message may be that young people take home from the movies, we can be sure that government speech directed to them in this or any other medium would be unlikely to make *Sweet Liberty*'s agenda of lighthearted rebelliousness its own.

The Electronic Soapbox

Dissatisfaction with the marketplace of ideas as it affects children is a special case. It turns on the recognition that children do not have the same legitimate right to autonomy as their elders. The very principle of an unfettered marketplace does not, therefore, directly apply to them. If we had faith that ours was a society in which families across the board consistently controlled their children and transmitted values across generations, then the marketplace of ideas might be sufficient, without government intervention. But that condition does not exist. So government intervention, government speech, was accepted into the lives of children long before any crisis in our perception of the marketplace arose as a result of AIDS.

But what about the marketplace of ideas for those who are not children, for those able to make important decisions about their lives? Here, the issues are more complex and more controversial. At the dawn of the AIDS crisis, the First Amendment tradition that had unfurled over the last fifty years was committed to process, with almost no concern for content. Each person was granted the right to speak his mind; the democratic marketplace was the place to sort out what was wise from what was foolish. This commitment to pluralism meant that we formally rejected the idea that there is some set of dominant messages that must issue from the combination of contesting voices. When the society seems to be functioning smoothly, questions about the mix of ideas in the marketplace are not asked. But when crisis strikes, results begin to take precedence over process, and analytical questions about the kind of information the citizenry is receiving become more dominant. AIDS is forcing us to look at the mix of ideas in the marketplace and at their impact on behavior and to ask some difficult questions: What proportion of the messages we receive reinforces ideas of social cohesion, respect for others, personal responsibility? If the mix is not appropriate, what should the government's role be in constructing and asserting symbols, in protecting the health and welfare of citizens through the definition and confirmation of community?

In eighteenth-century America, the mix of ideas in the marketplace was quite different from what it is today.[8] Notions of virtue and patriotism were much stronger, and the consumer engine that turns out most of the messages we receive today had not yet been constructed. Struggles for the minds of men and women were waged, but not by detergent companies and cereal manufacturers and travel agents and used-car salesmen. It is hard to overstate how different a marketplace of ideas our consumer society is from the one that existed when the First Amendment was written.

It is not only the mix of ideas that makes a difference but the technology behind them and the amount of money expended to assure that the ideas take hold. In other words, it is the architecture of the forum itself that determines what kinds of messages are sent and what kinds of government interventions are possible. The public park is no longer the locus for the shaping of consensus, and the soapbox as we once knew it hardly exists. As Owen Fiss has written, "There are no street corners, and the doctrinal edifice that seems . . . so glorious when we have the street corner speaker in mind is largely unresponsive to the conditions of modern society."[9] Now, we must worry about a marketplace that casually maintains and reinforces the existing power structure, through the prohibitive expense of entering the competition. This poses serious problems in democratic theory.

But from the perspective of a government that wishes to introduce a unifying message, one that is designed to affect behavior immediately, the evolved television forum, the modern electronic soapbox, has its virtues. Our society is once again a village, in some ways, one in which an electrifying message can make a commanding, immediate, and almost universal impact.

In the eighteenth century, neighboring countries and towns could have radically different religious theories and community habits, and geography was a sure way to absent oneself from a mainstream view that did not suit. Today, the pervasive nature of television has changed that. What an individual could accomplish through rhetoric in transforming a village can now be achieved in transforming a nation. This is a fundamental change in the structure of the forum.

Paradoxically, then, we have a marketplace where government is still restrained from interfering with private speakers, but one where it can intervene more effectively than ever before. We have a free-speech tradition which protects private speakers more than they have ever been protected, but we also have an array of speakers—shapers of the national psyche—who represent government or are more and more powerful, more and more like government in their influence and wealth, and who are often tied to government in the use of the electronic media as a federally licensed forum.

Governments have always been effective at dominating societies if they so chose. But modern forms of communication make dominance easier. It is no accident that television and radio stations are among the first targets of coup attempts. We generally recognize the propaganda that revolutionary governments abroad issue to the citizenry, but we are often unaware of the practice of propaganda at home. Yet the U.S. government has used telecommunications to achieve specific results from practically the birth of the industry. Propaganda during wartime is the most obvious case, and even in times of peace the Department of Defense is one of the nation's biggest advertisers, in its recruitment campaigns for the armed forces. From Roosevelt to Reagan, presidents have used the electronic media to defend policies and promote their own political philosophy to the nation.

One could argue that most of these uses of television or radio are different in content from a message about personal behavior and that they do not necessarily provide a precedent. But as

Mark Yudof has written: "The dangers posed by government advertisements may lie less in their explicit message than in the background messages. The agency involved and its officials are invariably portrayed as helpful and understanding, competent, and fully in control of a government apparatus that is successfully solving pressing societal problems."[10] Others have argued that government advertisements generally reflect a world in which problems are attributable to "individual carelessness, incapacity, bad luck, affliction, or fate."[11] In these public service announcements, "the solution to forest fires is individual care, not more forest rangers. America is kept beautiful by individuals picking up their litter, not by industries controlling their air and water pollution . . . Productivity increases depend on the worker, not on efficient management or improved technology."[12] One could conceive of an AIDS campaign which stressed individual responsibility, while avoiding the responsibility of the government to more adequately perform its role.

Thus, the architecture of the forum means that the government, during an AIDS crisis, has the tools to change attitudes more quickly and more thoroughly than would have been possible at a point of less comprehensive technology. And because there are fewer gatekeepers for the flood of information, the possibility exists for a central government to influence them more easily as well. Whether it can or should do so, whether the power to use the media ought to be deployed during a crisis, has a great deal to do with one's theory of the First Amendment and with one's commitment to pluralism. It is to that question of theory that I now turn.

The First Amendment in Transition

In the midst of a crisis, hysteria may compete with reason, and what passes for reason itself can become the product of the pressures of the day. The need for government to send forth a strong public health message in response to a growing threat and fear of AIDS may yield, at first, a voluntary acquiescence, a recognition that some form of public intervention is required. The danger is that we may lurch toward too strong a role for government speech that eventually changes our sense of the meaning of the First Amendment.

All this assumes, correctly I think, that interpretations of the First Amendment vary with the pressures of current conditions, and that each era fashions a set of practices concerning speech and culture that takes account of the imperatives of any given time. This does not mean that the First Amendment is meaningless. Far from it. Even if the Amendment itself did not exist as law, we would still have some set of principles or traditions that would embody the sense of the society about the meaning of free speech. In fact, societies might have stronger versions of the First Amendment on the books than we do, and yet free speech and individualism are stifled. On the other hand, some societies without a free-speech law are guided by much the same principles as those that guide us. The existence of the First Amendment to our Constitution is a factor—perhaps a very important one—in determining the communal settlement we have reached on these questions. But it is possible that the community's experiences have changed our interpretation of the First Amendment more than the First Amendment, per se, has changed the conduct of the society. The Amendment, under this theory, can be said to exist only to the extent that it continues to represent some deeply felt sense of the community.

I believe that the AIDS crisis is changing that deeply felt sense of the community about the meaning of free speech. More and more, the tendency seems to be toward an interpretation of the First Amendment as saying this: that the right of individuals to the free exchange of ideas without interference by the government (in the role of either censor or speaker) exists, and can only exist, in a society in which individuals are also subject to influence by other, compensating forces that promote values likely to guarantee the community's survival. These forces would include religious groups as well as families strong enough to integrate and balance the force of tradition with the urge toward creativity and dissent. Put another way, one might say that every community, to survive, must have a shared set of guidelines for public and private conduct. As long as these rules are being provided and enforced by social institutions other than a central government, then the government can afford to stand by quietly while these other social forces act and speak. But in the absence of strong institutions engaged in the transmission of values, governments must step in, especially in times of crisis, to ensure the society's survival.

Under this interpretation, rather than seeing the issue of free exercise of religion as separate from questions of free speech and free press, one might look at them as tightly connected. It is only by allowing religion to flourish, unencumbered, that a society could have the luxury of prohibiting Congress from abridging freedom of speech and of the press. Only in a society where traditional values could make their way, and where the sanctions available through religion and other strong family traditions were likely to occur, could government remove itself from the business of influencing values.

The late eighteenth century captures this combination. It was a period in which there were extraordinarily strong feelings about individual conduct, about the nature of expression, about the way in which values were stated, strengthened, and absorbed. Many of the communities that had been established in the colonies were basically about achieving and defending particular values. The influence of religion in accomplishing these purposes was intense; to say so in this summary fashion understates the impact of religion in shaping the American experience. The sanctions connected with private enforcement of religious values were intimidating indeed. In some ways they were more powerful, at least to those subject to them then, than much of what is in the armament of modern government. After all, religion often had denial of salvation as the ultimate enforcing tool, and imposition of the sanction did not rely on the unreliability of mere mortals. Religion did not require the buttressing impact of the state to ensure that its message was powerfully transmitted, but alliances with local governments to enforce community standards were often forged.

In this context, the First Amendment was not so much a monument to the principle of freedom from censorship of speech and press as it was a working rule for allocating the power to censor. To be sure, numerous contentious newspapers were mightily engaged in swaying public opinion during this period, and without question the First Amendment echoed vital concerns of the community about the right to political dissent. But more than that, the Amendment represented the firm determination by local government and religious institutions that the new and potentially dangerous force—the federal government—would not interfere in this most sensitive of human areas: the influencing of the community's values.

Personal freedom in this context was probably not exactly the bundle of attributes that many of us think of it as being now, a thing not only unencumbered by any government intervention but also striving to be free of organized nongovernmental forces in the society. Our current version of freedom can, only with difficulty, be reimagined in eighteenth-century terms to understand how the First Amendment was then perceived. Quite possibly, an important political message of those who framed the First Amendment and of the states in ratifying it was to tie the hands of the potentially powerful new federal government. Precluding the federal government from censorship was not necessarily part of a general policy of encouraging individual freedom and dissent as we now think of them. The question of proper levels of control would be left to other forces in the society.

A country that could adopt such a strong First Amendment must have had great confidence in the ability of its citizens, absent government, to preserve its mores. Just as some parts of the Constitution—the powers of the President, for example—rest on certain assumptions about checks and balances and the existence of the Congress and the Judicial Branch, the First Amendment rested on a particular vision of society in which there were checks and balances of another kind.

It would be foolhardy to believe that the First Amendment could function in twentieth-century America in the same way that it did in the eighteenth century. The forces that held sway two centuries ago—religion, local government, family—now have little power compared with their prior strength. The voices of new masters of cultural persuasion—the media and the advertisers, and perhaps the universities—have filled the vacuum in recent decades, yet even their influence pales in the face of the power our modern federal government could wield in shaping public opinion during a crisis, should it so choose. Calling upon its enormous bureaucracy and its extraordinary ability to control the electronic media, our central government is both capable of performing the role of cultural leader and poised to do so, should the crisis demand it.

If indeed the AIDS epidemic does lead to a reshaping of the moral values of our society, it would be a mistake—though one that many people will make—to attribute these changes solely to a rebirth of religious feeling in recent years and to organized religion's discovery of the power of television. Granted, in the 1970s and 80s organized religion has made itself more keenly felt than in the previous decade, pressing for more government support, or at least accommodation, and for wider definitions of free exercise of religion. The expansion of TV evangelism surprised many, and though a series of scandals certainly revealed some points of weakness, Christian fundamentalism clearly tapped into a strong force in American life during the Reagan years. Talk of strengthening the moral teaching of the young and of the reascendancy of religious influence became respectable in the White House. In this atmosphere, the Supreme Court held that Nativity scenes could be constructed at public expense and displayed on public ground, and seemed on the verge of approving some form of moment of silence in the public schools that might be the prelude to school prayer.

This resurgence of interest in religion suggests that, even prior to AIDS, the nation was becoming engaged in debate over the relationship between individual autonomy and the interests of the community. And because many religions offer theology-rooted solutions to the behavioral issues raised by AIDS, and draw on the power of television to communicate those values, it would be easy to credit religious forces with (or blame them for) the changes in values that we are likely to see in the wake of the AIDS epidemic. It is doubtful that religious forces alone have that kind of influence in a competitive marketplace of ideas. But an alliance between government and religious institutions speaking in one voice through the electronic media in the name of public health could become a formidable cultural presence indeed.

Behavior would undoubtedly yield to such verbal persuasion, but in the process we run the risk of relinquishing a set of principles that go deeper into our democratic traditions than sexual liberation and the celebration of self. What is at stake is the cherished, if perhaps out-moded, notion that the Constitution protects the individual's right to evaluate the pros and cons of behavior in an atmosphere that is free of government interference. If the AIDS crisis worsens, we may discover that we have lost faith in the ability of an unregulated marketplace to produce responsible attitudes and behavior; and, having no place else to turn, we may find ourselves relying more and more on the voice of government to articulate community values.

The perils that can ensue when government gets into the business of articulating values are illustrated in the AIDS context by a 1988 amendment introduced by Senator Jesse Helms. This amendment precluded the use of federal funds "to provide AIDS education, information, or prevention materials and activities that promote or encourage, directly or indirectly, homosexual activities." The Helms amendment became, instantly, a monument to the constraining hand of government. The legislation further encumbered the Centers for Disease Control, the Surgeon General, and others, curtailing the flexibility they needed to effectively describe conduct to be modified in light of the AIDS epidemic.[13]

Government speech, by its very definition, implies a specific set of messages—even a specific set of instructions about what messages are appropriate. What was heinous about the Helms amendment was the particular set of restrictions imposed (that is, the targeting of "homosexual activities"), the explicit and formal nature of the restrictions, and the linking of those restrictions to the use of any federal funds, even grants to private citizens. The Helms amendment is the most notorious example, in the AIDS context, of the entanglements that can follow from government speech, but it is not the only one. In 1985 the State of California created a review board which suggested that publicly developed materials use clinical or descriptive terms rather than slang or street language. In 1986 the Centers for Disease Control established guidelines to ensure that pamphlets and displays prepared under their aegis did not offend broad community standards; local panels were to avoid crossing the aesthetic or moral judgment of the ubiquitous "reasonable person." At all events, no material funded by the CDC could show explicitly the performance of safer sex or unsafe sex practices.

As it happened, the CDC guidelines inhibited flexibility, but not excessively. Yet the point remains that government speech, though sometimes necessary, has within it major dangers for democratic theory. If the government is speaking through its own officials and employees, it clearly controls the message—control is in the very nature of the enterprise. Indeed, in response to Surgeon General C. Everett Koop's frank Report on the Human Immunodeficiency Epidemic in 1986, then-Attorney General Edwin Meese announced sharply constraining official White House policy: "Any health information developed by the federal government that will be used for education should encourage responsible sexual behavior . . . based on fidelity, commitment, maturity, placing sexuality within the context of marriage . . . Any health information provided by the federal government that might be used in schools should teach that children should not engage in sex."[14] When the government is funding others, it will pick and choose those who can faithfully carry out the message that it wishes transmitted. Perhaps that is why we tolerate a Radio Free Europe only when we are attempting to propagandize or inform others, not ourselves.

New and competing interpretations of our constitutional protections arise not because of a brilliant discovery by a judge or a legal scholar but because of changes in the cultural context. Icons do not have one single meaning, and that is as true of the First Amendment as it is of the Statue of Liberty. The Amendment can mean many things simultaneously, and the intensity of any particular meaning can vary substantially over time and among those within a community. Yet, difficult as it is to identify, there usually is a predominant sense of meaning for the Amendment at any one time, a meaning that prevails in the literature, in common understanding, in the way in which the influence of the Amendment is felt.

To determine what that meaning is, we must turn to history, but not in the sense of studying history to determine what the framers "meant."[15] Rather, we must study the cultural context, and examine all the forces that affect speech and behavior at any particular time. In our own time, the AIDS crisis may rearticulate the story we tell ourselves about the First Amendment—about the proper relationship of private speech to government speech, and about the proper voice of government in shaping the culture. A society that interprets the First Amendment to celebrate the individual, to foster creativity by suppressing censorial urges—both governmental and nongovernmental—is different from a society that perceives, quite strongly, the need for a moral code that governs behavior. National crises—whether war, natural disasters, or massive threats to the public's health—can move the society from one vision of itself to another. This shift can already be sensed as we search about us for a proper response to the threat of AIDS.

part two

AIDS *and the Idea of Fairness*

One thing we know the constitution, the Equal Protection Clause in particular, cannot mean is that everyone is entitled to equal treatment by every law.

John Hart Ely, *Democracy and Distrust*, 1980

three

Discrimination at Society's Margin

AIDS has been a plague of blame and fear. It now promises to be a plague of unfairness, indifference, and discrimination. Increasingly, what characterizes a person with AIDS is not sexual orientation, or drug habits, or even age. Once the diseases associated with AIDS become dominant, abject poverty and dependence on the government and others for livelihood, medical care, and support become the new common denominators. AIDS has begun to impose extraordinary demands on a crumbling welfare system, creating reflections in some of our major institutions of what has been called "a new Calcutta."

In June 1988 Admiral James D. Watkins, chair of President Reagan's AIDS Commission, spoke about the federal government's sluggish response to the AIDS crisis, charging that a bloated bureaucracy had "acted as an impediment to a timely response." A report of the Institute of Medicine, part of the National Academy of Sciences, was even blunter: It condemned the "inequities in the entire United States health care system in relation to the uninsured and uninsurable, the plight of the poor in getting care, impecuniosity in funding for disease prevention, insufficient capabilities for the care outside of institutions and inadequate care for the chronically ill." Even the cautious *New York Times* wrote of a federal effort riven with prejudice.

The consequence of these burdens is an unfairness greater than the unfairness of AIDS itself, more than the mere freakishness of the epidemic. The cry, often subdued, is against institutionalized unfairness and discrimination. As the AIDS crisis in its second decade becomes more and more a matter of class and race, it becomes enmeshed with our constitutional notions of equal protection and the way we deal with inequities in the application of governmental power. Epidemiologists have the task of tracing the tracks of the virus, but all citizens must trace whether our response bears within it its own plague, a plague of discrimination.

Race, Class, and AIDS

Race is so fierce, so persevering, and so troublesome a theme in American history that it marks almost every category of life, almost every category of custom and law. There is precious little that escapes the burden of race. Race explains so much of what we are as a nation, our attitudes toward housing, education, voting patterns. Considerations of race help us understand otherwise mysterious demographic developments, such as where people live, where they go to school, how they are distributed in the workforce, how public transportation routes are designed. Things that start out neutral as to race, things as color-blind as a virus, quickly become enmeshed in the deepest structures of law, custom, behavior, and therefore race.

Race has played its role in the history of plague as well. In San Francisco in 1900, the Board of Health, fearful of bubonic plague, ordered a quarantine that meticulously circumscribed the movements of more than 10,000 people in the city's China-town, drawing lines that split blocks and curved around houses occupied by people of Chinese ancestry. Buildings and businesses within the quarantined district occupied by people who were not Chinese-American could maintain their livelihood and freely come and go. Doctors traditionally employed by Chinese residents were barred from entry. In a federal court case attacking the quarantine, the judge determined that the order—as well as being founded on wholly inadequate scientific evidence—operated "against the Chinese population only." It was administration of law "with an evil eye and an unequal hand."[1]

The AIDS virus does not discriminate on the basis of race, but the context in which it flourishes and the social response to it can. AIDS capitalizes on communities whose environmental and economic immune systems have been undone; it flourishes amid the scorn, isolation, and abandonment that already play substantially along lines of race in our society. In New York City, more than half of the adults with AIDS are African-Americans and Hispanics, largely as a consequence of the racial composition of intravenous drug users. Nine out of ten children who died in 1987 of AIDS in New York were minority children. The Centers for Disease Control has reported that a black child is fifteen times more likely to be born with AIDS than a white child.

As AIDS becomes a disease more and more of the poor, the African-American, and the Hispanic, traditional interest-group politics is likely to repeat itself in the politics of AIDS. Agencies established to serve the community as a whole will not pay attention to those of the underclass in proportion to their need. And special-interest groups rising to deal exclusively with the poor and minorities will have difficulty obtaining a significant share of public and philanthropic funds for their purposes. AIDS—like drug abuse, pregnancy among teenage girls, homicide among young men, unemployment, inadequate housing, and on and on—will become simply another affirmation of the existence of an underclass, and of our society's difficulty in achieving either the reality or the perception of equal opportunity for all citizens. The concern of government will be to control the virus so as to limit its spread to the more generalized population, rather than to defeat the disease within the underclass itself. If AIDS can be marginalized in this way—its devastation confined to the underclass—it will be marginalized in the collective mind, viewed as only another brutality among many that define the condition of that class in America.

The public is not yet at that stage. In fact, in the public mind, AIDS is not yet fully appreciated as a disease that so strongly implicates race and class. So much effort has gone into persuading us that AIDS threatens all—so as to change sexual behavior generally—that we have not focused sufficiently on the special interventions required among urban minorities. The question formulated by the media has been more whether AIDS will spread from the gay community to heterosexuals, less what its impact will be on the minority who are poor and black. Not right away, but in a reasonable time, strong, vocal organizations arose within the gay community to lobby for support, to change mores among its members, and to influence the external world's attitudes. Because the predominant group of those with AIDS in the minority community are people at its margin, particularly users of intravenous drugs, the environment for sustained championing, for arousing compassion, for influencing behavior has been far more limited. After all, AIDS among homosexuals resulted from conduct which, while thought to be deviant by a homophobic mainstream, was considered to be a celebration of self by many of those within the culture. No similar statement can be made about the use of intravenous drugs, minority or not.

Worse yet, in its relationships with those who establish the images that permeate the society, the urban minority poor are subjugated by old predators, prisoners of old ideas. Stereotypes of male sexuality and superiority remain strong in this culture. The high rate of teenage pregnancy is already a manifestation of failed education about caution in sexual behavior. Pregnancy rates calibrate the potential for the spread of AIDS among the young as graphically as they measure the birth of a new generation of the underclass.

AIDS is a matter of fact in urban shelters for the homeless, in city prisons, in the hospital emergency rooms where the poor, without their private doctors, must go for help. Yet, in the comfort of our living rooms, we debate the morality of distributing clean needles to intravenous drug users. In the safety of the legislative chamber, we condemn public information efforts that may strongly communicate preventive behaviors in clear and direct terms, our condemnation founded on hothouse sensitivities. Here is the possibility of a new form of discrimination, part of the plague of unfairness: an inability on the part of the government and the media to assert the zeal and the dedication adequately to aid prevention by revising the messages they target to this particularly vulnerable audience.

Some advertisers—Seagram, for example—have rejected advertising campaigns directed at a minority audience that trespass the zone of propriety considered appropriate for more universal television spots. But not all corporations have been so careful. In a television advertisement in 1987, black actor Billie Dee Williams, suave and masculine, wearing an elegant tuxedo and a red bow tie, handsomely fills the screen. The camera pans across his apartment: it is swank, the setting redolent of the potential for romance. A knock is heard at the door. Williams opens it to find a beautiful woman, proffering a six-pack of frosted Colt 45. The tag line is the refrain Colt 45 wants remembered: "It works every time." No study has determined whether there is a differential in sensitivity about persevering messages. But, nonetheless, here is an advertisement which implies the potential of an alcoholic beverage to produce fabulous and inspired sex, an ad directed at a largely black audience.

Minorities have been the target of advertising that is contrary to the interests of their health in other circumstances. As the rate of new cigarette smokers declined in recent years in the population as a whole, primarily owing to the success of public health messages from the Surgeon General, cigarette companies have focused their advertising on those groups where the prospects for increased smoking are better. Blacks, for example, have become a major demographic target for tobacco companies. This strategy may be viewed as strictly a marketing decision, not a moral one, in that no responsible person believes that any company is intentionally trying to increase the rate of lung disease among African-Americans, as opposed to other groups in the society. And yet, there is something about the decision, reflected in the fact that most corporate representatives will deny that it has been taken, which speaks ill of a society that allows it.

The case must be explored whether much programming, advertising, and music directed at a black population is less careful about encouraging behavioral change that increases the chance of avoiding AIDS. And though we may try to explain, justify, and gain an understanding of the complexities of this phenomenon, as with cigarette advertising that has a disadvantageous focus on one community, the outcome is unacceptable. Perhaps economic forces—what the marketplace will continue to accept—are simply more vigorous in requiring change where the mainstream is concerned. But if that accounts for the difference, then economic forces are not adequate to determine the course of the AIDS epidemic in the minority community. Those who program rock videos primarily for minority audiences and those who help to create other images that guide minority youths must send messages of caution as effective as those sent to the culture as a whole.

Public education about the risk of AIDS would seem to be the area of action least prone to discriminatory impact along the lines of race and income, but that is not the case. The capacity to educate rests on an existing structure—of schools, of families, of the other societal funnels through which public messages must pass. Without question, these structures are stronger for the mainstream than for the underclass.

The problem is not just one of preexisting poverty, or of school systems worn down by racial isolation, neglect, and despair. The problem is a failure, or unwillingness, to send a message that can be received and understood by the people most in need of it. In 1988 the Surgeon General sent to all households in the nation a clearly written, unambiguous Report on Acquired Immune Deficiency Syndrome. It is an excellent document, full of information, often blunt, but its unproven assumptions about communication leave one wondering whether the publication delivered an effective message to teenagers in urban ghettos who are at high lifetime risk for AIDS.

Television campaigns have been withdrawn and other educational efforts long delayed because of objections to the use of clear, if brutal, language and images that would immediately strike the consciousness of those to whom the message is addressed. This debate over niceties, this dance of decency, may have led to more effective public education for the middle class, but it has served to widen, not narrow, the gap between those who are informed about the dangers of AIDS and those who are not.

A brochure commissioned by the Centers for Disease Control, and produced by the advertising and public relations firm of Ogilvy and Mather, centered on the theme of "America Responds to AIDS." The brochure was designed to "prompt feelings of pride, patriotism, and reflect the American mosaic," according to a CDC memorandum. The brochure urged young persons to "discuss and understand life by your family's values." Teenagers are encouraged to say no to drugs and to sex. And adults are urged to find "a mutually faithful, single-partner relationship with an uninfected person, or at least be sure to reduce your risk by using a condom." Notwithstanding a special Congressional appropriation for distribution of the information, the Administration slowed its approval. "What exactly is it that people don't know?" asked a Reagan White House aide. "Is there a breathing American who doesn't know that you get AIDS from sex or a dirty needle? If there is, he probably is not the kind of person who reads his mail."[2]

This somewhat callous, though not inaccurate, observation highlights a major problem in targeting the underclass for a public education campaign. The task is a difficult one, requiring imaginative solutions. Brochures with the appearance of a sales pamphlet for surburban carwash discounts or new kitchen cabinets are suspect if the objective is to get information about AIDS to people at the margins of society. So far, the government's response has been restricted, and it leads one to ask what can possibly constitute fairness in the strategy to mitigate against the impact of AIDS, as it moves inexorably toward being an epidemic of the poor?

Addicts, Needles, and Quarantine

Race and poverty triangulate with AIDS not because of anything intrinsic about race, or about poverty, but because of the intersection of both of these with the fact of drug abuse. Among the 200,000 heroin addicts in New York City, half are thought to be infected. In the shooting galleries of the northeast corridor, hard-core addicts purchase drugs, rent needles and syringes, and often pay a person to jam heroin into their thigh. Blood is backed up into the syringe to ensure that the full effect of the dose is received. The needles, used over and over, allow the contaminated blood to be carried from one person to another. In this chain of poverty the deadly virus travels, linking the hopeless with each other in ways they cannot immediately fathom.

Intravenous drug users—already desperate, already somewhat segregated, somewhat under surveillance, already perceived as victims—are likely candidates for a break in the facade of civility and regard for individual rights that, thus far, has characterized the government's response to the AIDS crisis. The interventions we can foresee will be more significant than the refusal of doctors to treat patients, more consequential than the silent choices of medical students to attend nonurban hospitals and innkeepers to refuse guests.

The generally accepted view, prior to the current hysteria, was that society is already aggressively dealing with the problem of drug abuse. This view has been necessary because it is difficult for the community to face several of the possible explanations for the painful, sustained, and growing presence of drug abuse, even in the face of government action.

The realistic but unstated assessment may be that society does not have a productive place for those who have cut themselves off to exist in a drug culture. The jobs, the housing, the opportunities do not, in fact, exist. Under this view, there is a tacit recognition that rejection by the mainstream is rational. Race, too, plays a major part. As long as the majority community perceived drug abuse to be primarily a problem of African-Americans and Hispanics, the kinds and scope of action taken were limited. It is hard to admit to the possibility that the main-stream tolerates destruction at the margin. It would be tragic if the only major constraint on our tolerance of drug use prior to AIDS was fear that criminal conduct engaged in by addicts to raise funds for the purchase of drugs was a threat to the society as a whole. Now what we fear, too, is the spread of AIDS. And a measure of the relative importance of that new fear is the new enthusiasm we suddenly hear for massive drug-treatment programs.

The current recommendations to assist intravenous drug users are clearly transitional. Each day, in major cities, arrested and convicted intravenous drug users with AIDS are returned to the streets. Each day they are warned of the consequences of their actions, though the professionals involved know that few of these individuals actively control their conduct. The most ambitious proposals do not confront the reality of hard-core drug use, the despair, the recognition that early death is already the likely result of inadequate nourishment, inadequate shelter. This is a community where, at its core, death and disease have been a constant prior to AIDS. For a sufficient number, the recognition of the possibility of infecting others is not a compelling sanction.

Widely held postures about how to manage the drug crisis may be shattered by the AIDS crisis, but only after political leaders are willing to confront the need for gambles in the face of necessity. When a policy of distributing free, sterilized needles was first suggested by the director of public health in San Francisco, Mayor Diane Feinstein condemned the proposal as "a terrible and truly offensive idea."[3] Yet, slowly, the even more unthinkable idea of legalizing drugs may become palatable as discussion turns away from historic standards of conduct and toward the clear and present danger. Our impulse is always first toward restraint and compulsion; but then the rigor of seeking voluntary involvement by those who are infected or are at risk prevails. And then we must engage the nice calculus of determining what will make such voluntarism work.

A step in that direction was taken as the new federal administration took office: the liberalization of the availability of methadone, the synthetic narcotic which is thought to be a substitute for heroin. Reversing twenty-five years of restraint, the Food and Drug Administration has sought to make methadone available far more easily, not quite on demand but as close to that as might be considered seemly. Methadone is addictive, and those who use it as a substitute for heroin must be maintained in their habit; but it is not taken intravenously, so the hazard of continued spread is lessened. An army of the poor on methadone maintenance—some half million perhaps—is preferable to an army of the poor at hazard for AIDS. But it makes a mockery of the call for "treatment on demand." There is not the will, nor the funds, nor the expertise, nor the personnel to accomplish that goal.

So here we have a politically weak and needy community that is perceived to present a significant health risk to society, a community where individual action and the taking of personal responsibility are unrealistic solutions. The efficacy of treatment, given our state of knowledge, is low. Recidivism is frequent, and, indeed, the rate at which needles are shared, even by those in treatment, is far from known. Intravenous drug users often do not know that they can receive the virus from a person who looks healthy. They do not know that sterilization is effective or that boiling their needles does not harm them. They do not know that bleach can help kill the deadly virus. There is a threshold that will be crossed, if the AIDS crisis intensifies—some group, some place, will be first to be acted upon by category, the first group for whom individual rights will be suspended. Here will be the calls for quarantine and nonrelease from hospitals. The focus will be on constraining the victim, not on eliminating the supply of drugs. Drug abusers will be easy marks, for they will be assumed, probably correctly, to be exchanging dirty needles and engaging in prostitution, to be at high risk of infection and its transfer.

Given the extent of the epidemic among intravenous drug users, we cannot treat them with our normal laissez faire, laissez mourir, approach because the fiction of the isolation of the margin from the mainstream can no longer be sustained. Quietly permitting drug abuse while policing some of its external costs will no longer succeed as a strategy, and some difficult, disturbing choices about how to proceed will have to be made.

Children and Ostracism

Children with AIDS are also at the margin of society, often abandoned by their parents to hospitals or taken into foster homes. There is a silence about them; information is kept from friends of the children, from relatives of the foster parents. The stories recall the righteous Christians who hid Jews in occupied France or Holland. No one should know; no one should suspect.

The images of these children are of two kinds. These days, they are the pictures of infants with AIDS, in large part African-American or Hispanic, struggling to live, each one a burning tragedy. They do not speak. They are shown as illustrations of the consequence, by and large, of the involuntary passage of AIDS from mother to child, through drug abuse. Sad newspaper accounts tell of women in drug-using communities who are unable to alter their sexual practices because of opposition from men. Traditional sex roles change least in hard and desperate surroundings, where existing rituals may be much of what holds life together. And yet it is the avoidance of change which helps account for this poignant category of AIDS victims, a category now furthest from the general ken.

The other image is of an older child, often a hemophiliac, who was infected with the AIDS virus before the blood supply was screened, and whose fate is the cause of community concern. The child, at least in the media treatment of the subject, is usually white. The image here is of a Florida or Tennessee town or the outer boroughs of New York City, where public health experts work with school boards and the community to avoid immediate and brutal reaction and maintain the ongoing fabric of the school.

Fear of children is a new phenomenon, and it is testing ideas of fairness to which our society has professed devotion during the last two decades. As school boards allow children with AIDS to attend public school classes anonymously, parents demonstrate root apprehension about the safety of their children. Some take actions which, though spurred by concerns about health, will in fact perpetuate divisions along class and income lines. Those who can arrange, and afford, to place their children in an infection-free environment, or one that they believe is infection free, will do so. In causing a rethinking of decisions about schooling, AIDS will also alter patterns of friendships.

Fear of children may also halt the progress that has been made in mainstreaming children with handicaps, not because of any connection with AIDS but because we may rethink the relationship between the mainstream and those who are thought to be impaired in one way or another. The last two decades have seen a massive effort to alter perceptions about the way children learn, to promote the notion that there is mutual benefit for all in a system in which not all children are alike, in which children who are deaf, or blind, or otherwise impaired participate because they are functionally prepared to participate.

Peril exists even at the present level of apprehension about AIDS. Only with difficulty are qualities of democracy and equality learned, and even then they are fragile. Much of the effort to strengthen public education and the decades of work invested in reducing racial isolation and eliminating segregation were based on the theory that for a pluralistic society like ours to function, there must be more familiarity, more relationships, more interaction among the young across class, race, and income lines. It assumes that democratic leadership in the future comes from democratic activity among the young. It implies an atmosphere that is open, leading to toleration, exchange of ideas, and mutual respect. This feeling, vital to the political spirit, might be impeded by the AIDS crisis. It is already the case that informal, but real, quarantines are imposed on children with AIDS, those in hospitals and those outside who are known to have the disease. At home, aside from the particular injustices, children are learning lessons of shunning and rejection, lessons that took a generation to unlearn. In hospitals, families whose children are not infected insist on being in separate rooms, separate wards, separate buildings. Here rights are being removed not by official action but by the most effective and brutal action of them all, social ostracism, the silent, voluntary action of neighbors.

Mandatory Testing and the Workplace

Discrimination in employment is another arena where rights, arduously defined, may now be jeopardized. One important declaration of the society's commitment to the individual, especially over the last quarter century, has been the concentration on laws that limit or prohibit discrimination in hiring. These laws assert a conception of society in which individuals must be given their greatest opportunity to flower and be productive. Antidiscrimination laws have assaulted havens in the society that have been protected corners for privileged groups, havens defined by race or sex or other now-forbidden distinctions.

The changes that are reflected in these laws have been won at great cost. Much of the political energy spent in the period since 1950 has been to discredit and reduce or eliminate discrimination in the workplace—against people of color, against Jews, against women, against the elderly, against gays and lesbians. There have been marches in the streets, arrests, violence, and turmoil. Establishing principles of antidiscrimination as a symbol of the importance of the individual has been a wrenching national experience. It is not complete. Discrimination is so embedded in our collective psyche and in our individual attitudes that if it is to be reduced it must constantly be addressed. Public sanctions must always be clear and unequivocal. Each group at risk recognizes that selective discrimination is not a likely resting point for a community; for discrimination, once learned and practiced against one sector, is likely to manifest itself against another.

Now, as a consequence of the AIDS crisis, the first seemingly acceptable reappearance of discrimination is occurring. Employers are struggling with pressures to, at a minimum, require mandatory testing of prospective workers and institute measures that would isolate those who test positive for infection with the AIDS virus or, at a maximum, isolate all workers at high risk of infection. A summer 1987 issue of *Restaurant Management* magazine patiently details for its readership how the law limits the steps that can be taken. Then, reciting the precipitous fall-off in clientele when a restaurant is rumored to have workers infected with the AIDS virus, it recommends strongly that managers take effective action to rid their establishments of these employees.[4]

We ought to be fearful of an overwhelming and active discrimination reemerging in our national consciousness. Those who discriminate, who have strong prejudice, always have internally rational arguments for their position. They know why women should be excluded from corporate boards, why blacks cannot have positions of management in baseball. People who discriminate intensely do not think they are being irrational. In early 1988 it was reported that 40 percent of workers would worry about using the same cafeteria, and two-thirds the same toilets, as fellow workers infected with the AIDS virus. The possibility of an old and sweeping fear, almost always groundless, reemerges: fear of others, less openness to change. One of the greatest dangers of AIDS to the national consciousness is the threat to the principle, so arduously achieved, that baseless discrimination should be officially condemned and that private biases must not have public expression. This is why, perhaps, organizations so long dedicated to antidiscrimination actions have so fiercely objected to mandatory testing, and to any move that could be the first step toward a system of identification of, and action against, people infected with the AIDS virus.

Prisoners and Due Process

One evening, at the airport in Atlanta, waiting long hours for a plane to Florida, a young woman from the Louisiana countryside spoke of her brother, under criminal investigation for some offense in the small town where they grew up. He was going to flee from the United States, she said, fearing prison because of the risk of getting AIDS. Here was a new perception of prison, not for its official brutality, not for its loneliness, not for its punishment, but as a locus of disease.

Dealing with AIDS in prison means making odd calculations which must have existed before but which now have a special and ironic bite. Is it cruel and unusual punishment to convict a man with AIDS and condemn him to a prison? On the other hand, can a person escape the opprobrium of trial and conviction because of serious illness—in particular this one? More difficult, more irony-laden, is the question should persons with AIDS be released from prison even though they are part of the calculus of endangerment?

AIDS is an assault on a system that is already reeling with fatigue. To deal rationally with AIDS in prison is to assume an establishment that permits rationality to find a field of action. But overcrowding, marginal facilities, undertrained correctional personnel, populations at the racial and economic margins of society, sluggish processing of cases, an inequitable bail system—this is the arena in which the plague of AIDS takes place.

AIDS in prison forces us to confront fundamental questions about due process more frequently, often more openly, than has previously been true. It means examining whether it is absolutely necessary to have a defendant in the courtroom, or whether the person can appear via closed-circuit television. It means determining whether the lawyer has actually to be with the defendant or can appear on a split screen with the client. It means determining whether allowing disposable handcuffs, which distinguish prisoners with AIDS, additionally prejudices the judge, the court personnel, the jury, the probation board.

Questions about prisoners with AIDS define both how marginal prisons have become and how they have not become marginal enough: marginal because we have virtually surrendered the theory of rehabilitation, any idea that prison serves purposes other than punishment, retribution, the removal of danger from the streets; not marginal enough because there is commerce between the prison and the society at large. Prison fails to isolate permanently. And in the case of AIDS, the prison becomes, whether in myth or in fact, a place of special intensity, a place in which the virus gathers and then redistributes out into the world.

Confronted with the AIDS crisis, we roam through the social structure, looking for places to establish a system of supposed reason-based discrimination. In New York City, for example, because 90 percent of children born with AIDS are African-American or Hispanic, poor women in these groups who obtain services at some prenatal clinics are automatically tested for infection with the AIDS virus, and if they test positive, they are advised of the high likelihood that their fetus is infected and that, if born, their child may have a brief and painful life. Presented with the option to abort the fetus and have themselves sterilized, these women must decide, under circumstances that are psychologically oppressive, what to do. This approach is quite reasonable, in some respects, but hardly exemplary of free choice. In tacit ways, we are asking what right these women have to deliver sick babies into the world; we are revisiting schools to see what steps they can take to isolate AIDS children; we are determining under what circumstances hospitals can refuse admission and doctors can refuse to give care.

Now, already, hospitals have set aside rooms and whole wings where, like ancient lazarettos, only the sick and dying dwell. AIDS patients, two to a room, are rarely visited by those within or without the walls. In prisons, inmates with AIDS are pariahs. It is hard to provide enough education so that those in close quarters—prison guards, even companions in oppression—will consider the ill to be part of their bitter community.

Unless distinctions are meticulous, these actions are bad training for the national psyche. They will refresh the memory of old injuries and old practices and, perhaps, render them more legitimate again. But meticulousness is not a characteristic trait of crisis. And in times of perceived emergency, wholesale actions are taken even though those actions leave marks on our national character for generations.

four

The Vocabulary of Concern

These are harbingers of change, these new ways of thinking about children, about prisoners, about addicts, ultimately about race. Each is like the canary in the mine: a warning of danger in the environment. When the canary stopped singing, the miner knew that lethal gas threatened. A substantial task over the last half century has been to define the relationships between government and the most vulnerable of its citizens. As decades of interpretation have passed, the meanings have become more ornate, more refined, more detailed; expectations of constitutional protections have steadily increased. These were decades in which government laws and practices were scrutinized for potential discrimination against women as a class, against people of color, against the poor, against homosexuals. The question was how far this zeal would extend.

Now that zeal has slowed. It has slowed for many reasons, including the shifting membership of the United States Supreme Court. But the AIDS crisis is an aspect of the environment in which the judicial decisions, as well as many others, are made, in and out of government, and it promises to contribute, as a strong background circumstance, to the way we think about fairness.

When the debate, during the first decade of AIDS, has not been about the disease's scientific nature, the way in which the virus works, it has been about the fairness of the government's, and the popular, response. The key element of that discussion has been the struggle to define the way in which AIDS should be described, who is threatened, and why: Control the language and society's sense of what is fair follows. In this decade, not only have we had the language of stigma and blame, we have had the language of war and emergency, of plague, of equal protection, of utility and compassion. And now we have the language of race.

The Language of War

The vocabulary of war is already troublingly present in the discussion of AIDS, and it is a signal for attitudes that might come to prevail. The language of an embattled society, of an external threat and fallen heroes, of mobilization of government resources, of propaganda campaigns—all are indicators of a new vulnerability. In a health crisis, as in a military crisis, citizens anticipate that harsh and dramatic measures will need to be taken, measures that cannot immediately be explained and only crudely justified. Sacrifices may be in order, particularly by those who have the disease and may be the cause of its spread.

Equal protection of the laws and due process are guaranteed to all in the Fourteenth Amendment to the Constitution. But another policy—that in time of emergency government must be free to act—also has a long history, one that has prevailed over the competing niceties of particular constitutional constraints. War is the most obvious time when the existence of the nation is clearly put to the test and when the needs of the society as a whole must be put ahead of individual rights and protections. But other emergencies, if they are extensive, can also muffle debate about constitutional formalities and encourage the taking of decisive action, even if that action involves the suspension of rights. The question is whether the AIDS epidemic will become such a serious threat that, in the public's mind, it takes on the stature of war.

Democratically selected authority may lurch to delegate much of its power to experts, as happened in Camus' *The Plague*, when the Prefect of Oran, faced with the need to impose extraordinary measures, turned to the doctors and asked for their professional declaration that an epidemic existed. Only the entire Congress has the power to declare war, but a single public health official can declare an epidemic. And just as it is hard to challenge the general as he establishes strategy in battle, so it will be hard to second-guess the assumptions or recommendations of a public health official charged with strategy at the time of crisis. As under martial law, one expects that orders about public health measures will come crackling out, some comprehensible, others not.

There may be pressures to fabricate answers even though answers do not exist. If an enemy can be defined, even roughly, retribution may be demanded. In post-liberation France, at the end of 1944, one of the resistance papers demanded "a thousand heads and five thousands arrests" to wipe out the score against the collaborationists. Due process was not a popular idea. In her *Paris Journal*, Janet Flanner pointed out that the "eloquent, calm pleas against repeating what in France's Revolutionary days was called Le Terreur have been made, usually by good citizens not in mourning."[1] To satisfy a public demand for action should the AIDS crisis intensify, the cheapest place to take from will be the realm of individual rights.

More than once, as the specter of quarantine has floated in the national consciousness, the memory of the exercise of federal power in World War II has been renewed. Those were days, too, of fear and potential danger. The response, then, to a fear of subversion mixed with prejudice was to round up Japanese-Americans and take them to internment camps, with no due process at all. And in *Korematsu v. United States*, 1944, the United States Supreme Court sanctioned military response.[2]

That decision demonstrates how, in times of war, like times of public health crisis, the actions of government become clothed with an unusual inviolability. The problem, unresolved, is how to establish limits to the actions of government when it is impressed with what seems to be its fundamental responsibility to ensure survival. Of course, the Constitution applies to actions of the government at all times: The trap, as the Japanese internship cases so dramatically and painfully demonstrated, is that we seem destined, weakly so, to accept as constitutional much that is seen as necessary at the moment.

Korematsu was an America citizen of Japanese descent who had remained in his home, contrary to military orders authorized by Congress. Those orders compelled all persons, with no inquiry into their loyalty, to report to "Assembly Centers," as part of a process virtually imprisoning them. Justice Black, upholding the conviction of Mr. Korematsu, demonstrated the support for authority that often conquers all during times of perceived crisis. For him, under the circumstances, it was impossible to reject as unfounded the judgment of the military authorities and of Congress.

"We cannot say," he wrote, "that the war-making branches of the Government did not have ground for believing that in a critical hour such persons could not readily be isolated and separately dealt with, and constituted a menace to the national defense and safety, which demanded that prompt and adequate measures be taken to guard against it." The impossibility of "immediate segregation"—in the case of the internship, the separation of the loyal from the disloyal—justified upholding a broad order. "Hardships are part of war, and war is an aggregation of hardships." "When under conditions of modern warfare our shores are threatened by hostile forces, the power to protect must be commensurate with the threatened danger."[3]

In his concurrence, Justice Frankfurter was wary of making the Constitution "an instrument for dialectic subtleties not reasonably to be attributed to the hard-headed Framers." "To talk about a military order that expresses an allowable judgment of war needs by those entrusted with the duty of conducting war as an 'unconstitutional order' is to suffuse a part of the Constitution with an atmosphere of unconstitutionality."[4]

Even the dissenters shared in this rhetoric. Justice Roberts dissented on the grounds that the Court had severely misstated the circumstances and extent of the government's action. But he agreed that "the civil authorities must often resort to the expedient of excluding citizens temporarily from a locality." "The . . . removal of persons from the area where a pestilence has broken out," he pointed out, "is a familiar example." Justice Jackson, though forcefully dissenting, acknowledged that "the armed services must protect a society, not merely its Constitution." In time of war, "no court can require a commander . . . to act as a reasonable man."[5]

The crisis of epidemic is a natural substitute for the crisis of war. In a forerunner to *Korematsu, Hirabayashi v. United States,* Justice Douglas concurred in upholding a curfew, using words that are hauntingly resilient as we face a possible public health emergency. "Peacetime procedures," he said, "do not necessarily fit wartime needs." And though the number of disloyal people, like the number of those who may pass the AIDS virus, was a tiny percentage of those who were subject to the order, that was not the end of the cause. "The sorting process might indeed be as time-consuming whether those who were disloyal or suspect constituted nine or ninety-nine per cent . . . But where the peril is great and the time is short, temporary treatment on a group basis may be the only practicable expedient whatever the ultimate percentage of those who are detained for cause."[6]

The *Korematsu* decision is ritually discredited today. It has been condemned, vilified, separated out as a creature of another time and the hysteria of war. The Commission on Wartime Relocation and Internment of Civilians has concluded that the internment far exceeded any military necessity, and Congress has voted reparations to those interned. But the haunting feeling is that *Korematsu* is not a fluke. When those in power determine that draconian action is necessary to offset public peril, when there is popular support for that position, then the Constitution will establish a standard but not one that will necessarily and immediately prevail. The lesson of the Japanese-American internship cases is that it can happen here, that there are circumstances in which individuals otherwise entitled to equal protection will see those rights diminished because of a deemed national necessity.

Law becomes a gracious song that can be sung when it is possible to sing it but abandoned when it is not. Necessity is the test of the society's mode of dedication to the rule of law, both what occurs in a time of fear and the circumstances in which fear takes over. It is decisions like *Korematsu* that give the lie to formalism, that call into question how valid the formal statement of the law might be. And it is circumstances like the AIDS crisis that measure when emergency makes its entrance and when the careful architecture of normal moments is temporarily dismantled.

We are not in the time of *Korematsu*, not yet, and there is room for tribute that Admiral Watkins and Surgeon General Koop had broader visions than General DeWitt. The consequence is a challenge to look in the other direction, to determine how to be effective and humane, how to implement a strong public health campaign while avoiding the damaging harms of reinforcing prejudice. We seem to have learned, partly from *Korematsu*, that it is necessary to scrutinize government action to determine whether invidious discrimination exists, and, if it does, whether it accidentally or purposefully hurts those outside the power structure and, as a result, is especially unfair.

The Language of Plague

The metaphor of plague has permeated the AIDS era. Indeed, early on, AIDS was called a "gay plague," confirming and burnishing the idea that the AIDS epidemic was rooted among the homosexual risk group and, moreover, that a moral stigma was attached to its existence.

The journalist Richard Goldstein has written that many illnesses "transform their victims into a stigmatized class, but AIDS is the first epidemic to take stigmatized classes and make them into victims."[7] Stigma has a contagion separate from that of the infection; the interaction of the epidemiology of both requires attention. The general public seeks to read the data of incidence narrowly, to hold the disease to the homosexual community. In that sense, stigma is used as a protective device to maintain the normalness of their lives and expectations. If stigma dominates consciousness, the danger is that the public turns more strongly against the groups at risk than against the disease.

Diseases of the past have intimidating names, names like the Black Death, that call forth all sorts of associations, of class and caste and perhaps especially of remoteness of culture. Stark differences between cultures, and from century to century, mean that there are few constant rules about the social consequences of disease. Yet historically important occasions of mass illness have almost always changed personal behavior and altered the character and texture of societies. That may well be what distinguishes those diseases that are, in common language, plagues: As a result of something more severe than epidemic alone, these events scrape against the basic relationships in the society. Traditional patterns of doing things are overturned. Fear or demand for action changes relationships among individuals and may change, as well, the nature of the state.

Plagues bend history. Diseases were a factor in the conquest of Mexico by the Spanish, in the saving of Canada for England during America's Revolutionary War, in the decimation of those anciently native to the continent during the settling of the West. Severe and brutal disease helps explain the failure of Athens to defeat Sparta, the vulnerability of the Roman army to attacks from Asia, and the shift of power away from the Mediterranean coastlands in the sixth century. What is remarkable, in retrospect, is how unusual, perhaps how illusory, the last four decades since the polio epidemic have been, at least in the West, in the absence of contagion.

There are diseases of our time that have been far more widespread than AIDS, have had a higher mortality rate, have arisen just as suddenly, but are not thought of as plagues and do not have the overbearing social consequence that AIDS seems to have. During the last decade, the hepatitis B virus shared a number of the characteristics of AIDS. It passed from person to person through blood, it was more dangerous to doctors and other professionals, it was often fatal, it affected large numbers of people. Until a vaccine was discovered recently, a discovery which yielded a Nobel Prize for its research team, there was no known cure, and even less public attention.[8]

Each great epidemic has its own peculiar history, dependent on the structure of society in its time, the real and perceived nature of the disease, and what people think can be done to prevent or assuage its dread consequences. Always important is the religious and moral sense of the community, how it divides causation between the natural and supernatural, and what it considered to be the very message of the disease. In Muslim orthodoxy, plague has been an act of mercy sent by Allah, to be accepted, not resisted. The idea of taking preventive actions was itself heretical. In Christian medieval Europe, plague might have been divinely sent, but it was with a message that had to be interpreted, as were the plagues sent upon the head of Pharaoh to let the people of Israel go. Disease did not impose a duty of fatalism. Blame was to be found, but there were also the obligations of charity; as a consequence, it was not always thought inconsistent with faith to take steps to try to prevent or contain the scourge.

Plague is a convergence of disease and circumstance in a way that yields substantial change in a community. Because deeply held religious feelings have for so long affected the way people have thought of themselves and their circumstances, plague often has had a moral connotation, as if it were visited upon mankind in retribution for wrongdoing or to demonstrate divine power. This moral and religious connotation persists. Calling a disease a plague still bears the suggestion, especially where there is an accessible object for blame, that there is a moral as well as a scientific basis for its existence. Cyprian, Bishop of Carthage, wrote in 251 A.D. that "the just are called to refresh-

ment, the unjust are carried off to torture; —How suitable, how
necessary it is that this plague and pestilence, which seems
horrible and deadly, searches out the justice of each and every
one and examines the minds of the human race."[9] For some
indigenous people of the New World, plague would be a cause
for conversion, for explaining supernaturally what became a
matter of great political consequence, namely, that their con-
querors were unharmed while they were decimated by diseases.
Blame is also a way of distinguishing the observer from the
source of fear. And, in a time of fear, there is an avalanche of
blame that often seeks out those who are already at the margins
of society. In 1831, after an outbreak of cholera in Leeds, a
milliner wrote to his brother: "It appears to me that the Lord is
scourging us as a nation for our multiplied sins . . . it ravages
more especially the drunkards and the sabbath breakers."[10]
There was a widespread increase in churchgoing, as one historian has noted, "so that an avenging God could clearly distinguish between the moral and the immoral."[11]

The language of plague builds in its own notion of fairness,
and a disturbing one. The reference to plague reminds us of
those myths and stories when a society is collectively punished
and searches for a cause within to extirpate, a particular person
or group to blame. David Richards has brilliantly attacked the
use of plague language to discuss AIDS on the grounds that the
idea of moral plague "has familiarly been used as a tool of
cultural purification of outcast heretics to traditional moral values," and that now it is a convenient metaphor for "what is
essentially a kind of heresy persecution of homosexuals as moral
heretics to the family."[12] Without meticulous distinctions, the
use of plague language mars our understanding of AIDS and
can detract, too greatly, from the less ambiguous medical and
public health models for care.

The Language of Equal Protection

The language of equal protection provides a compelling vocabulary—one that gives voice to rights, not merely persuasion. In

a society that has not been generous with absolute constitutional entitlements—we do not have a constitutional right to education, to work, to medical care, even to vote—we have resorted to a language that measures the inequities of fortune. If a government that does not have a constitutional duty to provide health benefits decides nevertheless to do so, it must ensure that they are provided without discrimination. We are, however, still confused about the meaning of equality—about the measurement and treatment of differences, about which inequalities are acceptable and which are attributable to government.

Our commitment to pluralism further complicates the principle of nondiscrimination. In some versions of its conception, the Fourteenth Amendment's goal was relatively clear: to bring to former slaves the rights held by white citizens. Almost immediately, though, the language of equal protection was captured in the service of businesses seeking shelter from state regulation. Only in the late twentieth-century has the language of equal protection been used to question the pace and distribution of federal bounty. Simpler models of equal protection have given way to more complex forms, now often legislated, in which the society opens itself to examination for discrimination on the basis of gender, alienage, poverty, sexual orientation, and handicap. Redefining equal protection under law to incorporate this increasingly pluralistic vision of the society is difficult, because the standards by which we determine when a particular group has been disfavored by the government's action or failure to act are no longer clear-cut. Now, even the determination that there *is* a norm may be questionable.

Most critiques of the federal government have berated it for its minimal response to the AIDS crisis. This was the implication of the reports of the National Academy of Sciences and of the President's AIDS Commission. Adequate money for research and education was not requested by the federal government. When it was obtained, it was not immediately spent. Rather than a sense of urgency, there was perhaps a strategy of neglect. Politics among federal institutions—specifically between the

National Institutes of Health and the Centers for Disease Control—were a significant factor in muffling the impact of the event on the federal government. The Food and Drug Administration was sluggish in permitting the use of new drugs. These charges raised questions concerning more than aimlessness and bureaucratic mismanagement. A breach of fairness was alleged, linked to a failure of haste because of the nature of the victims. The question has been raised whether a scorned subgroup—people with AIDS or, more to the point, gays with AIDS—was ignored and subjected to a pattern of government discrimination, and whether more would have been done had the disease struck, with equal devastation, a more popular group.

The constitutional issue of equal protection is complex, though the term is often invoked. We do not live in a system in which some constitutional talisman tells us the "right" method of distributing wealth or health. Ours is, for better or for worse, a society that *presumes*, indeed thrives on, inequities that arise not out of the denial of opportunity itself but out of the differences in the way opportunity is seized. We know that the Constitution does not mean that every person will fare equally well. Yet, when we evaluate a course of government action—at least according to constitutional traditions—we must ask whether a higher level of scrutiny ought to be exercised because of the very nature of the risk groups affected by the AIDS crisis.

If AIDS were a disease that struck only a racial minority, we would have the machinery to see if, within it, there was careless regulation that fulfilled discriminatory impulses rather than proper legislative needs. But the group first affected by government policy concerning AIDS—gays—is not defined by race. Yet it is the kind of group where the wisdom of Justice Stone is instantly relevant: Those at risk of obtaining AIDS are subject to the kind of "prejudice against discrete and insular minorities" that tends to affect the operation of political processes in a manner contrary to our basic values.[13] The consequence of being so disfavored a group is the kind of prejudice, as John Hart Ely has put it in *Democracy and Distrust*, that provides the natural majority with "a common motive to invade the rights of other citizens."[14] We should be particularly suspicious when a government approach disadvantages a group which, for long-standing reasons, those in control of the legislative process may seek to injure.

And now that race is so deeply implicated in the course of AIDS, the dangers are compounded. The task, as Ely has put it, is "uncovering official attempts to inflict inequality for its own sake—to treat a group worse not in the service of some overriding social goal but largely for the sake of simply disadvantaging its members."[15]

Lethargy, inaction, bureaucratic impediments—these are the hardest of governmental forms to bring to traditional constitutional analysis. Slowness in the face of crisis can be criminal, in a popular sense, but it may be quite constitutional. In the AIDS crisis, the slowness had, at the least, an impact on a disfavored group and, at most, designedly so. That is why, instinctively, we think of denial of equal protection. But discovering animus or impact is not the only analytic obstacle. In thinking about unfairness, we start with a model, fictional but useful, of a government minimal in its functions, one which has less of a responsibility to worry about jobs, or shelter, or adequate food on the table. In a world in which the government's responsibilities are few, the idea of equal protection is easy to conceptualize: What government does, it should do evenhandedly.

But we are far from such a model. We turn to government in the AIDS crisis, as in so much else, to cause research to be done, to provide the leadership in both science and education. After complexity enters, almost any government action can be defined as discriminatory to someone. A government that builds no roads seems to be harming no one disproportionately. As soon as a road is proposed and built, some are advantaged and some are disadvantaged. Those along the side of the road see their property increase in value; they are brought into the mainstream. Those who are not in the path of progress may complain that their government is not acting equally with respect to them.

The Supreme Court was extraordinarily subtle when, in 1886, in the case of *Yick Wo v. Hopkins*, it struck down a San Francisco regulation affecting laundries.[16] There, a statute neutral on its face, prohibiting the use of wooden drying equipment, was being used almost exclusively to put Chinese laundries out of business. *Yick Wo*'s principle—that we must examine in some detail the structure and operation of government to determine whether it is unconstitutionally discriminatory—is applicable to the AIDS crisis. The governance of the AIDS crisis encapsulates how needful we are of central government services, particularly in an emergency, how dependent we are on government initiative, and how reaction or nonreaction by government can have disproportionate impact among citizens and groups. Yet the difficulties in attending to questions of equity in our complex society are enormous.

If we restrict the inquiry just to our health care system, how would one measure the propriety of research into heart disease or cancer as opposed to research into the causes of AIDS? There might be fruitless and detailed examination of the nature of the patient population at the National Institutes of Health to determine whether patterns of discrimination in patient admissions exist. One could ask whether basic research programs in medicine should focus on illnesses that plague racial minorities as much as illnesses that afflict the mainstream. But these are questions that are almost impossible to answer. Even seeking to answer them may be perceived as an untoward intervention in the scientific enterprise. A strong belief in the importance of unencumbered basic science, of encouraging research without too specific an eye on the outcome, is the centerpiece of modern thought about scientific progress. How can one apply equal protection principles to free inquiry?

Courts have taken over prison systems and educational districts in order to remedy the consequences of discrimination. But these are harsh steps in a democracy. It was a thunderous act, at the time, for the United States Supreme Court, in 1954, to hold that a scheme of separate public schools was inherently unequal. That strained the capability of the courts and the nation almost to the breaking point. In the AIDS crisis, unevenness of impact from the government's actions is much less explicit, the questions much more subtle. Issues of budget and subconscious intention involve comparisons that have rarely been made. Discrimination in the government's strategy toward AIDS, if it exists, would require the courts, if they accept the invitation, to become much more detailed auditors of strategy, much more subtle examiners of intention and impact than they have ever been before.

A further obstacle is that we are dealing here with undeclared rights, not the denial of a proclaimed constitutional entitlement like the right to a jury trial. While we have a system in which it is wrong to discriminate in the distribution of medical services, there is no absolute constitutional right to public medical care, or to a federal research program, or to health insurance, or to a job. And except when Congress or a state legislature is in an extraordinary pique, rarely does legislation show unconstitutionality or unconstitutional intent on its face. Even when Louisiana, in the 1930s, under the spell of the Long family, wished to strike out at newspapers that did not toe the party line, the Legislature masked its venom by imposing a tax based on newspaper circulation. Conveniently, the test swept within its net all the detested newspapers, while those papers that supported the Long family were, except for one, excluded.

As a society using a vocabulary of judgment more keen and powerful even than that of the Courts, we have to look both at the terms of a statute and at its impact to determine whether the government divides up the world in ways that should arouse our suspicion that something wrong, in an unconstitutional sense, is going on. What hurts those with a high risk of getting AIDS are failures on the part of government to take the steps necessary to hasten research or provide experimental drugs or alleviate poverty or cause an environment in which some of the root causes for drug abuse are not present. What is the vocabulary of judgment? Oddly, government acts within its political bounds if, as Ely puts it, "insensitive as they may often seem to some of us," budgeting decisions stem not "from a sadistic desire to keep the miserable in their state of misery, or a stereotypical generalization about their characteristics, but rather from a reluctance to raise the taxes needed" to support them.[17] Usually government will be able immediately to translate its decisions into these constitutionally innocent terms. Oppressive unconstitutional intent may be present, but it is always buried within layers of other motivations and seeming necessities. That is why it is painfully difficult to brandish effectively the language of equal protection when faced with the mysteries of bureaucracy and the anguish of competing priorities.

The Language of Pragmatism

Ultimately, the best prospect for fairness arises from a general public desire to meet the challenge of AIDS, to support strong leadership, to allocate adequate resources, to rethink institutions and practices in light of pressing needs. So far, in the AIDS epidemic, the language of pragmatism has set the boundaries of fairness, defeating harsh emotion. Pragmatism has found its home, most securely, in what Ronald Bayer has called the voluntarist perspective, the recognized need for willing involvement by those at risk, those infected, and those with full-fledged AIDS.[18]

In almost every instance when mandatory testing was rejected, when discrimination was sanctioned, even when the closing of bathhouses was extensively and torturously debated, government action was most effectively opposed on pragmatic grounds. Experts have been pitted against politicians in the struggle to determine the right balance between self-generated participation and state coercion. Sometimes the seemingly easy way has been followed, as in the ultimately overexpensive mandatory screening policy affecting all who seek a marriage license in Illinois. The federal government has imposed mandatory testing in the military, the Job Corps, and the Foreign Service.

But, by and large, the pragmatic appeal of voluntarism has been a buffer to many proposals for compulsion. Initial proposals for a broad program of mandatory testing—for all hospital admissions, for example—gave way to a consensus for broadly available, highly supported voluntary testing. The sharp edge of state compulsion was removed because of the sense that the most important benefit was reaching and reeducating those at risk and helping to find those who were infected but did not show the symptoms of AIDS.

The tendency to pass laws to control behavior is typical of any circumstance in which a legislator can appear thoughtful by enshrining a prohibition in law. Some states have already modified their laws to permit the quarantine of carriers of the AIDS virus who engage in behavior that might lead to the spread of the disease. Colorado, for example, authorizes public health officials to order infected persons to stop behavior that is dangerous to others and, if they fail, to restrict them in some way. Florida has made it a crime for a carrier to engage in sexual relations without disclosing the risk. Tennessee makes it a crime for an infected person to donate blood. Louisiana makes it a crime to intentionally expose another to the risk of AIDS. Nevada makes it a crime to practice prostitution after a positive test for antibodies to the AIDS virus. Federal statutes have been considered that would criminalize the donation of blood or semen or organs by a person who knows he or she has tested positive or is even a member of a high-risk group.

Are these statutes useful beyond the satisfaction of the moment? Are they discriminatory? In certain cases, such as assuring that donated blood is free of the AIDS virus, criminal injunctions are not sufficient: The community has to test the donated blood. Yet there is a certain satisfaction, a certain fulfillment, in establishing through the criminal law system a code of behavior that outlines what is no longer acceptable, even if the criminal law does not achieve the proper level of deterrence.

These statutes are a substitute for other forms of progress. If there were sufficient medical advances—the discovery of a vaccine—then the need to seek comfort through the relatively nonfunctional mode of criminal law would not be so pressing. The 1988 Report of the President's AIDS Commission took a thoroughly utilitarian view of the law. The principal question asked was whether a proposed measure would contribute to the containment of the epidemic, not whether it would fulfill a communal taste for justice. If more testing is likely to occur in a voluntary mode, then mandatory testing is disfavored. If the articulation of norms of behavior through criminal law increases paranoia and reduces cooperation, then imposing a criminal law should be reconsidered.

Utilitarianism was the basis for the Commission's recommendation that the government pass a federal statute that would make discrimination against people infected with the AIDS virus unlawful. If the AIDS epidemic is to be contained, they reasoned, then persons with AIDS must be willing to come forward, and persons at risk must be willing to undergo testing. Cooperation is the key to management of the crisis. And for that to occur, those who stand to lose from the potential for discrimination must be encouraged to participate.

This is a logical but difficult mode of thinking. It does not ask whether conduct—in this case, discrimination against people infected with the AIDS virus—is wrong, or outside the acceptable limits of polity. The AIDS Commission sought to build a consensus for federal antidiscrimination legislation almost wholly on the grounds that the practical goal of containment should take priority over these questions of morality. There are virtues in this kind of pragmatism. But people need to fight prejudice on the basis of justice and basic human values—because the argument from utilitarianism may sometimes fail.

Perhaps the very fact that the AIDS Commission's recommendation in favor of antidiscrimination legislation has not made its way into law tells us that we do not yet imagine ourselves sufficiently at war with the AIDS virus to require such a practical approach. But it may be a premonition of something more forbidding: As the demography of AIDS shifts, as those infected become increasingly poor and minority, perhaps we are less prepared to rely on the voluntarist perspective. Pragmatic objections to harsh public actions may lose their political force. In the first decade, public health officials, primarily the Surgeon General, made progress in reconceiving AIDS as a general health hazard and not as a narrow stigmatizing plague. As the second decade of AIDS begins, that progress is itself at risk. We are still free enough of the pressures of the moment that we can stand back and ask not just whether a given measure is immediately useful in the effort against this virus but whether it squares with our notions of justice. As drug abuse, race, and poverty become more dominant in the discourse about AIDS, as personal catastrophe turns into a social and financial abyss, the luxury of debate, the politics of voluntarism, and the exactness of minimal intervention all may become victims of the times.

part three

AIDS *and a Crisis of Confidence*

The confident assumption that medicine is a science and not an art, the product of steady and
sometimes spectacular advances in drugs and technology, has been shaken by a disease that recalls
the days when tuberculosis and polio killed young
patients while doctors watched. All medicine can
do now is postpone death.

Washington Post, January 15, 1988

five

Lost Mastery

Until very recently, much of what we have been encouraged to desire and expect in our lives is constant improvement in our station, unending technological innovation, a clean, comfortable, worry-free existence. The advertisers' image of the sleek, luxurious automobile, insulated, safe, nothing out of place, symbolized what we thought the modern world ought to be like. This vision of technology in the service of freedom, comfort, and efficiency—expressed in the 1939 World's Fair—is still all about us: in the futuristic freeways of southern California, in the calm, friendly skies of jet travel, in the VCRs, the VDTs, the HDTVs. Technology has been an instrument of liberation, releasing people from life's drudgeries and accountabilities. Reading is replaced by television, arithmetic is replaced by calculating machines, letters are replaced by preprinted greeting cards, fossil-fuel pollution is replaced by nuclear energy. And if we find ourselves feeling unaccountably anxious or empty, our bad moods can be ameliorated by medication. Whatever is disagreeable about life can be conquered technologically.

The technological fixes that are most effective are self-executing, automatic, not dependent on human choice. We seek a birth control pill that works for a month so that day-to-day vigilance is not necessary. We yearn for a similar solution for AIDS, one that will not depend on that scarce commodity, the exercise of individual responsibility.

We still do not have a vaccine to prevent the spread of AIDS or a drug to cure it. AIDS, perhaps as cancer has before it, is slowly eating away at our faith in the authority of medicine and, because of the intricate dependence of medical advances on government support, may lead us eventually to question the capacity of the state to meet a national crisis. A world in which disease governs more than man is a world for religion, not law.

Technological setbacks in the past have already shaken our long-term optimism. Three Mile Island, the bureaucratic mismanagement that led to the Challenger disaster, the toxic pollution that is the downside of improved materials, our inability to deal with nuclear waste and other detritus of a bloated civilization—all these are the background for our apprehension about the prospects for blocking the spread of the epidemic.

Will an alliance of science and government solve the AIDS crisis? Will technological expertise, backed by all the resources government can muster, somehow come through and save the day? If our faith in scientific progress falters in the face of the AIDS crisis, will our faith in the state also wither? In the long absence of a technological fix, what resources can we call upon to cope with the threat of infection, and with the thousands of people already dying of disease? In raising these questions, AIDS embodies not just a constitutional crisis but a crisis of national confidence as well.

Autonomy in the Bionic Society

One of the last frontiers for the realization of technological advance is the human body. Our society has become obsessed with the notion of perfectability in that most personal of spheres, one's own physical self. We have come to believe that, through proper diet, exercise, and new biomedical advances, disease and disability can be avoided or at least repaired. Reaching old age in excellent health is assumed to be practically a birthright of the American middle class.

Through cosmetic surgery, we can pursue the goal of appearing forever young. Through reproductive biotechnology, we have the goal of demystifying and controlling the nature and occasion of birth. Prior to the AIDS epidemic, when we thought of medicine, we no longer were haunted by visions of nineteenth-century death wards, of helplessness and despair; we focused instead on triple-bypass heart surgery, the survival of tiny premature infants, kidney transplants, laser surgery. Medicine in our time has become not just a product of modern society, or a piece of it; it leads and, in a way, justifies modernity.

This attitude toward biotechnology molds the sense of the individual in society. If we think of the bionic man and woman of 1970s television, we see, conjured up, individuals who could surmount almost anything, for whom personal danger existed but only in the absence of complex corrective science. Here was the difference between the Superman myth and the Bionic Man myth: One was the creation of another planet, the other was the product of human accomplishment. But what is common to the two myths is that physical invulnerability permits heroic acts; it permits a person to undertake far more than would otherwise be possible. Modern medicine gives a little piece of the myth of invulnerability to everyman.

How we think about the capabilities of science and medicine determines how strong the myth of our invulnerability is, and the strength of that sense of invulnerability in part determines how we conduct our lives. In the area of sexual behavior, the discovery of the effect of penicillin on syphilis and the invention of the birth control pill probably had more to do with changes in our attitudes toward permissible sexual conduct than all the social movements, advertising campaigns, and religious reforms combined. Science lowered the cost to the community of what was once called promiscuity, and our legal system has responded to this change in the community's sense of right and wrong. The whole idea of removing legal sanctions from so-called victimless crimes arises from the notion that the society should give wide berth to those actions by consenting adults in which no additional costs to the community accrue. On the surface, medical science has seemingly expanded the zone of individuality because it has made it appear that personal conduct that would have clearly had external consequences now lies within the realm of immunity and invulnerability. Indeed, though large-scale medicine is a complex social undertaking, its effect has been to emphasize the idea that the individual can act outside the community.

But when epidemic strikes, it is clearer that what one person does has an implication for his fellow citizens. The fatal illnesses of recent memory are different from AIDS: they are solitary. Cancer and heart disease are about survival in a polluted, stressful, sedentary environment. They are not about the danger of one person to another. Something echoes from the more distant past in the way AIDS makes us potentially secret instruments of affliction against our fellows. AIDS partakes of a consciousness that existed in the time of influenza in 1918, when in some cities all were required to wear face masks; or in the time of leprosy, when laws were passed forbidding lepers to touch public buildings. It is a consciousness that existed when people feared public pools because of the possibility of contracting polio.

At present—before the discovery of a magic-bullet cure—AIDS has reintroduced the idea that personal acts have consequences. We recognize a stronger relationship between how individuals behave and how society functions than we supposed to have been the case during the last two decades. Indeed, the activity that, prior to AIDS, sparked the most fervent defense of the notion that government should not create victimless crimes was sexual acts among consenting adults; yet, ironically, it was specifically consensual sexual intercourse, primarily unprotected anal intercourse, that turned out to yield social consequences of the greatest magnitude.

The libertarian principle that government intervention is untoward where acts have no social consequences is still strongly supported. But the realm of the principle narrows as our faith in the ability of medical science to obliterate AIDS and similar tragedies dims. The existence of a disease should not necessarily be the moment for a paradigm shift. But because medical science cannot erase the physical and financial consequences to the community of these personal human interactions, one result of AIDS may be that all libertarian claims are perceived with greater suspicion and circumspection. We may be less willing to believe, arrogantly, that our science has permitted us to foresee most long-term ramifications of our behavior.

Testing the Mechanistic Model of Disease

The notion that humankind can master disease and gain some measure of control over death has its roots in the Scientific Revolution of the seventeenth century. The world-view of the Middle Ages had presumed that the natural world was at the mercy of supernatural forces. The massive plagues of the four-teenth and fifteenth centuries only served to reinforce this religious belief that people are not in charge of their own destiny. In pointing out the thin line that separates societies from chaos, plague was a reminder of the fragile nature of earthly civilizations.

A reawakening of interest in science led to the view—essential to modernity—that recurring and regular sequences of events govern life and can be described and plotted in a quantitative way. Medicine in particular gained ascendancy by showing that an understanding of the natural world leads to power to control it. Here, even at this early moment, was the notion of mechanical medicine, of the human body as a machine whose internal workings could be understood and regulated; here was the source of the twentieth-century assumption that when the parts of the human machine are fully understood, anything that is working improperly can be fixed, and eventually mechanical breakdowns can be prevented from occurring. In its task of mapping the structures and functions of the body, the budding science of medicine was as spirited and triumphant as Renaissance explorers had been in the discovery of new lands.

At the beginning of the nineteenth century, unhealthy urban

areas typical of industrialization yielded new masses of sick and, as a consequence, huge hospitals to house them. Doctors became more organized as a medical profession; and, unlike fifty years before, patients, especially in the urban hospitals, were increasingly of the working class, inferior in social status to the doctors who treated them. With this change, patients were less and less possessors of individual symptoms and increasingly statistics. While in earlier years the patient contributed greatly to determining the nature of his or her disease, now it was the doctor, primarily, who classified, who adjusted cases by category. This was the foundation of modern public medicine, in which all concepts are converted into applications, all ailments turned into objective diseases. Disease became an entity almost separate from doctor and patient. At this time, also, a theory of causation became more concrete. Ill health was traced to the malfunctioning of a particular part of the body.

From the second half of the nineteenth century to the present, laboratory medicine has flourished. More and more, medicine has become one with the natural sciences in its use of the experimental method. The focus on the cell as the basic unit of the body led, in the twentieth century, to new vaccines, to sulfa drugs and antibiotics, and to an understanding of the role of DNA. The current era of genetic engineering can be seen as the full blossom of the mechanistic view of the body.

For many honest optimists, AIDS is to be yet another chapter in the march of medicine as science: urgent and exciting, "first and last a scientific research matter," as Lewis Thomas has said, "only to be solved by basic investigation in good laboratories."[1] The armies of science are at the ready, with new partnerships among branches of inquiry already taking place as a consequence of the imperatives of AIDS. Given enough time, enough funds, enough imagination, scientific medicine will yield the answer, according to this view. Conquering AIDS is not something that the lay public should concern itself with, except as a transitional phenomenon. The progress of mankind, the way in which society is organized, these can be considered free of concern about illness and its consequences. Those can be handled by medicine, which, in its evolved, scientific way, is a near-perfect machine.

The fervent wish for a technological solution to AIDS, a cure, a vaccine, is reflected in the frequent press accounts of new developments by researchers around the world seeking to understand how AIDS works and then to construct an approach to vitiating its impact. In Stockholm, at the 1988 World Health Organization AIDS Conference, thousands of scientists gathered, their tentative researched conclusions reflected in a forest of wooden paddles by which each sought attention, forlorn pieces in a monstrous puzzle. With each assertion, discovery, claim, fear, the public's attitude toward the possibility of another medical conquest is shaped. "We will learn how to destroy this virus," a young doctor has written. "Until then, I will make sure that for both myself and my patients, there is room for quiet triumphs and private victories."[2]

But there is a deeper, more pessimistic perspective on the history of medicine and technology. AIDS, as the Nobel laureate Joshua Lederberg has written, is but a recent chapter in the ongoing struggle among macroparasites and microparasites. For Lederberg, the planet is one giant test tube in which interactions between all parts of being are constantly occurring over time. There is no dominance. The idea of the human at a permanent pinnacle is arrogant, destined to yield confusion and disappointments. "We are complacent to trust that Nature is benign," Lederberg has said. "We are arrogant to assert that we have the means to except ourselves from the competition."[3] The idea that humans can conquer all microbes, that they can maintain permanent dominance in this complex interplay, is a vain projection of the person-centeredness of our view of the universe.

Lederberg sees the world through his test tube, in which he watches and enacts "the wipeout of populations on a gigantic scale, and of course recognizes that this is an unremitting process in nature." He echoes the historian William McNeill that while humankind has asserted its control over the environment in many ways, making man the most significant enemy of man, there still exist "our principal competitors for dominion . . . the microbes: the viruses, bacteria and parasites. They remain an interminable threat to our survival."[4] Human life is forever vulnerable to the massive changes that occur when relationships between parasite and host, or between any two competing species, are upset. In the test tube, these changes occur in an instant. For mankind, time and change are of a different order, or at least we perceive it to be so, and the puzzle is that we cannot know with any exactitude what the shape of our time and change in the test tube of the planet will be.

The implications for science and medicine must be viewed, in the long term, with pessimism, according to this view. AIDS is a reminder of the powerful, unrelenting rhythm of natural processes. It is the rumble of a grim past, mocking modern advances and the claims to order of a legal system. Even advances such as the expansion of antibiotics have within themselves the seeds of their own obsolescence, because of microbes' ability ever to mutate and become resistant.

We fool ourselves into thinking that control in the developed nations can quarantine illness incubated in other parts of the globe. As Lederberg puts it, "Our neglect of infectious disease in the poor majority of the world is not just a humanitarian disgrace; it leaves unchecked the seeds of our parochial infection." Biology and medicine, Lederberg suggests, can solve problem after problem, but in the longer range, it is doubtful that they can totally change the wall of fact that is the relationship between humanity and microbes.[5]

For Lederberg, the relevant history for understanding AIDS is the history of the earth, the ongoing competition for survival. For Thomas, the relevant history is much more the history of mankind itself and the relationship between medicine and science. "Cascades of surprise from laboratories all round the world," Thomas has written, "will almost surely lead to novel therapeutic and preventive approaches that cannot be predicted at the present time."[6] It is in this history of medicine, with its prospect for control, that the answer to AIDS can be found.

Lederberg believes that the contest is much in doubt. We may not yet know the virus that causes AIDS; if we do know it, there is the possibility that it may mutate. Awful though it may sound, the possibility cannot be dismissed that the virus could change into one that can be transported through the air, so that the entire way we think about the epidemiology of AIDS may be altered. For Thomas, these are concerns, but concerns that will be taken care of in the course of scientific research: "No human disease is any longer so strange a mystery that its underlying mechanism cannot be understood, or got at." The contest is one only of time, and funds.

Challenging the American Way of Death

In the not-so-ancient past, people had little control over the time or circumstances of death. So long as disease was uncontrollable, death lurked nearby and had to be considered as always possible. This classic sense of death—as not within our control, as something which often happens inexplicably, unjustly, randomly, as something which smites great nations with horrible plagues—is an essential part of the myth, memory, and customs of humankind. Perhaps it is our changed view of death that alone accounts for changed views of religion, of redemption, of an afterlife.

Our present view of death—in the absence of a perilous, massively threatening disease—is that it can be postponed. Death has become, in Lewis Thomas's phrase, a sort of failure of living rather than an inevitable event. Death occurs as a result of violence, the kind that appears in the movies or on the 11 o'clock news, not as something which is a significant and constant part of one's lifetime. Merely to die, in the modern mind, is not to have lived properly.

Medicine and prosperity have been heroic in achieving ways of circumventing death. In one generation, we have taken steps through the transplantation of organs, indeed their very manufacture, to suggest that we may ultimately control when death can occur. This change in our view of death is one of the hallmarks of our time, a dramatic aspect of what it means to be a person in modern Western society. Certainly, the very material change in life expectancy since the beginning of the century has strong implications in demography and in the organization of the state. But more than that, the idea that we are in charge, that the combination of resources plus science can help determine, quite substantially, the length of life, has wrought extraordinary internal psychological change. Not for us the myth of the Fates, spinning, measuring, cutting, and controlling human destiny.

The emergence of AIDS is shocking to us, in part, because it reintroduces the ancient idea of death as being outside of human control. We read accounts in the newspapers, now not the body counts of Vietnam but the actual and potential body counts of disease. This is a kind of death new to many, one that is a particularly ugly possibility because, like war, it reaches those in the prime of their lives, often at the height of their creative gifts. This reassertion of death has already affected our art, theater, and literature and begun to reshape a part of the Western psyche. Death and disease, as with people in centuries past, may again become part of our lives.

Arien Mack has written of the relationship of the art of great disease to its times: "Images of people suffering from bubonic plague, which had once uniformly displayed human helplessness and the comforting intervention of saints, were slowly superseded by representations of purposeful (though often frustrating) action to organize a social response to mass illness."[7] This evolution is confounded, somewhat, in the AIDS crisis, as imagery reverts to helplessness and away from the confidence that the potential for control—governmental or scientific rather than divine intervention—exists.

Renaissance artists found in St. Sebastian a figure whom they could mold as a response to the ravages of epidemic disease. In their paintings, St. Sebastian is shown with eyes heaven-bound, bearing the darts and arrows which now allegorically bore the poison of the bubonic plague. One great fresco shows the figure of God throwing destructive bolts, with Christ and the Virgin Mary kneeling and imploring Him not to inflict the scourge on mankind. In the nineteenth century it is Napoleon, saint-like and heroic but also an emperor ruling on earth, who is shown in a monumental painting, *Pest House at Jaffa,* by Baron Gros, defying the weight of mythology, actually touching the sores of those dying from disease. By the twentieth century, when the human role in resisting the spread of disease had become dominant, artists were enlisted in more modern propaganda, urging, often through poster art, individual actions that conformed to social needs. As propaganda, art was in the service of the machinery of control.

In the last few years, visual artists have sought to affect the individual and public response to AIDS. Rage, protest, and escalating anger—these have been a preeminent reaction by artists to government policy seen as insufficiently urgent, characterized by inadequate funding, clogged approval of new drugs, and halting research. But another artistic contribution has been exhibition after exhibition of photography, often in bleak black and white, showing AIDS patients isolated and alone. An art of endurance, it shows no promise, little hope. "Until That Last Breath" was the title of an installation of such photographs on the subject of women with AIDS at the New Museum in New York. By documenting progressive illness and death, this style dramatized the failure of collective human action, and prized the solitary sufferer, by showing the irrelevance of context. It is an art form for the benefit of artists as well as viewers, a form of therapy that allows them "to come to terms with the terrible sense of pain and loss that is part of death."[8] This is not Napoleon touching the sores of the dying, nor is it St. Sebastian interposed symbolically to receive the bolts of disease. It is an art form some have criticized as relying on pity and fear when those emotions are a weak base for the dream of scientific triumph or the recognition of the value of individual defiance and struggle. But the art form reflects the weakness that occurs when the illusion of control and confidence is in peril.

The AIDS crisis provides ample opportunity, too ample, for us to review our attitude toward the conditions of individual choice that surround death and the act of dying. Here is the ultimate question concerning the status of the individual. Should the individual be allowed to decide the moment and circumstances of his or her own death, or should the physician be required, despite the clear intention of the patient to the contrary, to maintain and prolong life as long as technology and resources will allow?

This was one of the most poignant of the national debates of the 1980s. The radical improvement in the life-sustaining capability of medical technology has raised these questions about medical decisions and patient choices from abstract philosophy to daily necessity. The questions range from resuscitation to withholding care, including medication, and allowing death to occur "naturally." What control over these steps—prior to the critical moment—should be given over to the patient? How much discretion should those who are administering care have to override the patient's stated wishes, or to determine themselves that no further effort is justified?

AIDS poses these questions in ways that are difficult for the individual and society to confront. To say that AIDS is almost always fatal is to ignore important subtleties that affect moral and ethical as well as legal realities. Death is a certainty for all of us. At various stages of our lives, we are all inevitably in a contest with death, taking whatever measures we can to slow or speed its inevitable arrival. We take risks, we avoid risks. We also leave room for the deus ex machina, the miracle, the cure, the delaying possibility, the chance of beating the odds.

In these respects, men and women with AIDS may be different in degree from the rest of the community. Perhaps they have a greater right to serve as subjects for experimental drugs, and to determine when treatment should desist. As one tribute to these concerns, a consensus has emerged for hastening the availability of new drugs. And since AIDS patients may face extraordinary ravages, extraordinary pain, the humiliation and difficulty of cumbersome medical procedures, they may press the point that they ought to control their own lives, and that part of exercising that control is the right to determine when death should no longer be deferred.

Much is at stake in terms of widely and deeply held religious belief. Many tribunals, including the New York State Commission on Death and Dying and the New Jersey Supreme Court, have emphasized the importance of patient choice, absent the AIDS crisis, or with AIDS only a large shadow over their deliberations. The question is whether the pressure of AIDS, its particular pattern, its prospect of severe illness and impending mortality, will alter the line any further. Will it result in practices that yield patient control over decisions to die at an earlier point than could be foreseen in even recent pronouncements?

The Limitations of Bureaucracy and Expertise

Prior to AIDS, we moderns had become so confident of our mastery in science and technology, particularly as they apply to medicine, that we lost sight of how relevant a factor the history of disease has been in determining not just our sense of individuality but also our sense of community. In the shaping of modern Europe, the actions of generals and kings in the fourteenth and fifteenth centuries pale in comparison with the long and cyclical exposure of communities to mortal plague.

Think of a disease that twice or several times within the memory of a generation sweeps through a community, rapidly causing almost a third of its members to die. Think of a disease that removes, through death, a substantial number of leaders and, as well, those who produced goods, who were depended on for the necessities of life. The Black Plague shook society. It affected the power and ideology of the Church, altered the economy, changed the face of medicine, forcefully isolated individuals, and, some historians believe, demonstrated the limits of elaborate hierarchies to function at a time of crisis.

In times of epidemic, the struggle for order over disorder, for a sense of control as opposed to a sense of fear and anxiety, engages not just physicians and biomedical researchers but government officials empowered to make policy in order to protect the public health. In our society, the premise of the public health profession and its use of law is that control of disease is possible—that we are capable as a society of defining a management approach that will minimize contagion through proper levels of public expenditure, legislation, manipulation, coercion.

Yet there is something in the AIDS epidemic of lost mastery. We sense a limit not only in the ability of science to conquer this disease at the biological level but a limit in the ability of government to function in a scientific way—to weigh and balance complexities, to articulate criteria and choose a path among the political requisites that is logical and rational.

We had hoped to get a sense of control from the eagerly awaited final report of the President's AIDS Commission. But despite the thoroughness of this document, it has virtually disappeared from public discourse. The President's Commission on the Human Immunodeficiency Syndrome, as it was clumsily called, and the detailed, lengthy document it published in June of 1988 were expected to be important events in the evolution of a national policy on AIDS. Appointed by then President Reagan, the Commission was, at its outset, hopelessly split, a kind of cartoon extension of extreme views about AIDS, including homophobia and distrust of government. In a way, the original Commission reflected the confusion of the nation as a whole, perhaps also its innocence. Only after the resignation of its first chair and the appointment of Admiral James Watkins to replace him did a consistent, overarching, and detailed picture of a national policy concerning AIDS take shape. This picture, described in the final report, was delivered to the White House with much prepublication fanfare and with a precision befitting a military chairman.

The general acceptance of virtually all its conclusions by commission members with sharply differing views of society was a great accomplishment; the comprehensiveness of the report was an achievement; the willingness to articulate some basic concerns about American society that are implicated in the AIDS crisis was daring. Still, there is something desperately wistful about the report, perhaps a silent acknowledgment that its major cries will go unheard, an unspoken recognition that the social context in which government must function is so extraordinarily complex, unruly, even corrupt that any set of recommendations—and the report abounds in recommendations— sounds somewhat hollow.

The discussion of government policy with respect to drug use is an example, though actions in the early Bush administration (such as the more extended availability of methadone) give one hope. The report concludes that "the nation's ability to control the course of the HIV epidemic depends greatly on our ability to control the problem of intravenous drug abuse." And, as a consequence, a ten-year strategy on drug abuse is needed. The recommendations have an all-too-familiar ring. And because they are like so many that have been made before, the sense of failure arises almost as the words are read: more availabililty of treatment, more federal funds, more local funds, model demonstration programs that are community based, help with the families of drug abusers, provision of risk reduction information, political and community leadership. The report asks that drug abusers "take responsibility for their own well-being and that all aspects of government do more to curb the entry of drugs from abroad and the production of drugs domestically." Enormously ambitious, these recommendations seem wholly without footing in the gnarled and ugly collection of facts that leads to the existence of drug abuse on a wide scale in the United States. The report urges an extremely aggressive policy without adequately acknowledging the vast and complex interrelationships that make it difficult for the nation to alter its drug-use policies. The report may correctly tie the AIDS epidemic to a need for changes in drug policy, but the report could establish no authority for change and makes little compelling case for change beyond that which existed in the absence of AIDS.

One of the hallmarks of the report was its plea for federal legislation that would protect those with AIDS or infected with the AIDS virus from discrimination. And yet here, as with its recommendations concerning drug use, the Commission gave the illusion of coping with the complexities of the subject, but in fact did not do so. The urging was largely on functional grounds, namely, that in the absence of discrimination it would be hard to encourage those with the possibility of the virus to come forward and seek help. And without that cooperation, control of the epidemic would be more difficult. And yet the complex issues involved in extending federal authority were only rudimentarily discussed. To the extent that federal law would bind institutions and employers who obtained federal financial assistance, existing federal law might be sufficient. To the extent that law would be extended to include all who engaged in interstate commerce, then a massive shift in responsibility, including prohibitions on discrimination against all who are handicapped, would probably be required. It was unclear why AIDS would be a sufficient lever even for what might well be a suitable reordering of the mode of government intervention in hiring and other practices.

Persistently, the AIDS Commission's report underscored, even unwittingly, complexities of overreliance on government regulation and government practices. The report was a textbook example of ways in which the modern state, like modern medicine, has become the perceived repository and authority for the solution of problems. Expectations have risen dramatically in the last half century. Charged with maintaining military dominion in large parts of the world, the state is now also expected to provide education, health care, and employment whenever other institutions in the society default on their responsibility to do so.

Our modern society searches for a science of law just as it

searches for a science of medicine—for a rationality, for rules grounded in scientific principles, for appropriate legal remedies to harsh and troublesome problems. In the criminal law, for example, the movement toward parole and probation was founded on scientific attitudes toward human behavior, on the belief that we could determine when something like rehabilitation was possible and could construct the circumstances in which the prospect of improvement would be most likely to take place. Debates about capital punishment often turned on scientific data concerning the deterrent value of the death penalty, the scientific view being that such a punishment might be warranted if its utility could be proved and, most certainly, could not be justified if its utility was in question.

Indeed, to a large extent, the modern state operates on faith in expertise. From the 1930s forward, when Roosevelt refashioned government by increasing the functions of administrative agencies, it was expertise that was to carry the day. Congress delegated power to agencies because of their growing expertise. Courts deferred to these agencies because of their expertise. A reshaping of law had occurred, in large part because of the presumed preeminence of expertise as a road to progress.

AIDS becomes part of the questioning of government expertise. The Food and Drug Administration is mocked for its bureaucratic deliberativeness in testing the effectiveness of drugs. The health care delivery system is mocked because of the delay in finding alternatives to expensive hospital care. The educational bureaucracy is mocked for its inability to provide instruction to young people, particularly the very poor, about the risks of unprotected sexual intercourse. As each agency or part of government becomes touched with the need to cope with the complexities of AIDS, there is a new sense of ordeal.

The advocates of people with AIDS strike a resonant chord as they seek more directness, more simplicity, more responsiveness and compassion. Critics, even before AIDS, were faulting the shift of power away from Congress and elected officials as undemocratic. They decried the shift in adjudication from juries and lay judges to commissions and panels of "experts." These critics contested the idea that a more ideal society is attainable through scientific and technological expertise than through the good sense of ordinary citizens and their chosen representatives.

AIDS is a harsh teacher, bringing us a painful tutorial in history and civics that was previously omitted from the curriculum of our time. It has returned death and illness to the vocabulary of everyday life, mocking common aspirations and assumptions about ever-longer life and the power of people over their fate. As the epidemic calls into question our ideal of health, it also undermines our faith in the protective power of wealth and expertise that, for fifty years, has been grounded in the modern progressive state. We are forced in the presence of AIDS to acknowledge the thin veneer of civility that orders our relations one with another, and perhaps to treasure those connections all the more. Instructed by AIDS in the fragility of civilization, we are moved to its articulate defense, even as we are thrown back on ourselves.

six

Searching for a New Paradigm

An abiding legacy of the AIDS epidemic in America will be its effect on the relationship between the individual and the community. No similar period of intense, widespread introspection and reexamination of how private life should be conducted has occurred since the 1960s. Then, the inquiry was an open, expansive, celebratory one, a breaking of constraints, a seeking to establish worlds without limits. Now, in a context of fear and necessity, of haunting reminders of the tenuousness of survival, our ties with the past and with each other are being restored.

Paradoxically, the very idea of the modern state—with its technology and science—is often justified by the opportunity it provides for individual expression, growth, and freedom. Indeed, countering the centripetal force of government bureaucracy the last half century is the emphasis, at least in the language of the law, on the strengthening of the individual. The tension in the midst of the society's encounter with AIDS is how to harmonize these two traditions: the need to emphasize individual responsibility at the same time that centralized government action is required to minimize the disease's impact. Each area covered in this book—the reordering of speech and behavior, the ensuring of fairness, the questioning of progress in science and medicine—yield a different sense of the relationship between individual and government.

Allegiance to the Individual in the Law

How the individual is perceived in the society is the very essence, the fundamental building block, of much of our legal system. Only in light of that fact do the stakes involved as a consequence of AIDS become comprehensible. Our twentieth-century idea of privacy itself, expanding on historic doctrines shielding people from unlawful searches, grew from a sense that protection of the individual from government intrusion is one of the most important constitutional goals. This notion of privacy nourished constitutional decisions that protected a woman's right to determine whether or not to have an abortion, forbade Connecticut from enforcing a ban on the use of contraceptives, and impeded state enforcement of antipornography laws against persons reading or viewing obscene material in their homes.[1]

Allegiance to the individual transformed the law of conscientious objection. Historically, the exemption was permitted only to those whose objection was based on a religious belief, with a specific religion being required as a source and underpinning for the objection. But in the 1960s, the Court broadened the doctrine to include deeply felt individual moral objections that were the functional, but secular, equivalent of the religiously founded concern. This interpretation flowed from a sense that the individual's commitment, rather than his connection to an organized religion, ought to be the basis of the right to conscientious objection.[2]

The expansion of protections for suspects and defendants in criminal prosecutions and trials also grew out of a new respect for the individual's freedom, one that goes far beyond the familiar cavil that it is better for a hundred guilty men to be set free than for one innocent man to be held in prison. The laborious dictates of the *Miranda* case, which instruct the police to warn suspects of their right to remain silent and their right to have counsel, reflects the philosophy that the fragile individual is most at risk, most subject to sudden destruction, when faced with the organized power of the state.[3]

The law's approach to the family has increasingly emphasized the primacy of the individual over that of the family unit. The notion that the state should establish conditions for the dissolution of a marriage has been more and more rejected. Now it is two individuals, not the community, who determine, practically speaking, whether a divorce will occur. Adultery as a specified and limited ground for divorce is inconsistent with the modern idea that the state should not concern itself with ranking personal behavior. Family adjudications are increasingly concerned with facts, not moral claims, with descriptive evaluations rather than prescriptive conclusions.[4] A legal system has been evolving that tends to a kind of efficiency, allowing the widest possible range of individual actions to be taken. Any moral statement contained in law begins to bear the burden that it must be defended. Why should law require people to remain married who do not wish to? Why should law preclude married people from having sexual relations outside marriage? Why should law prescribe the gender of spouses or their sexual orientation? Why should law preclude the trafficking in children?[5]

This attitude in law goes beyond the family. It puts in question restrictions imposed by government on the way a corporation designs the architecture of shareholder rights in the company. An expanded and strengthened metaphor of rights is used to limit the power of the community to impose zoning barriers. It weakens the power of the Food and Drug Administration to restrain the testing and sale of experimental potions. The metaphor of rights makes it more difficult to comprehend any legislative regime that gives community values primacy over individual freedom: laws that protect the family farm system from bankruptcy, the American economy from imports, children from obscene or indecent programming, neighborhoods from gentrification and redevelopment, and the reservations of Native Americans from the termination and dissolution of common land into parcels for individuals.

All throughout the law there are examples of this movement, over the last half century, to prize the individual, to establish an order that will encourage individual autonomy and freedom.

Further, the way we think about law is repeated in the way we think about other aspects of our lives. Emphasis on the individual is at the foundation of our economic system. We vaunt consumer choice as the hallmark of our way of life. And, of course, the sanctity of the secret ballot and the historic trend toward more direct representation demonstrates our commitment to individual choice as the mainstay of our political system. The autonomous and free individual is at the heart of how we see ourselves personally, how we see ourselves as economic men and women, and how we see ourselves as citizens.

Balancing Community Values on a Tilted Arc

This increasingly central aspect of the individual oddly parallels changes in public art of recent times. The sculptures that are in our parks, the murals in our public places, once told stories and sought a strong relationship to their audience. Today, public art is largely about art itself, about the importance of creativity. Richard Serra's *Tilted Arc* was a massive, abstract Cor-Ten plate commissioned by the United States for the Federal Plaza in New York City which came under bitter attack from many of those who worked in the vicinity and which was eventually taken down. They thought that the work too assertively proclaimed itself, with insufficient sensitivity to the needs and visual aspirations of the community in which the work was placed. Serra's defense was in large part based on the First Amendment—the right, he claimed, of an artist to express his individuality. Having commissioned and installed this site-specific work, the government could do little, if anything, to remove it, he unsuccessfully argued. Removal would be an infringement of Serra's individual rights as an artist, a form of censorship. This would be true despite the temporary or even enduring reaction of the neighboring community.[6]

This sense of sculpture in public places is far different from that of its antecedents. If one thinks of the monuments to the Civil War, the statues of solitary soldiers, the classic generals on horseback, other allegorical and massive sculptures, the intent was didactic, highly moralistic, narrative in a way that communicated with a popular vocabulary.

Serra's *Tilted Arc* forces us to ask how in our modern society we are going to balance the focus on individualism and autonomy with a sense of community and responsibility. And just this clash of values that confronts us with respect to Serra's work of art is now confronting us as we deal with individual rights in the face of the AIDS crisis. In each instance analysis demands the nimble shifting between the aspirations of the individual and those of the community. We are practiced in a mode of thinking, characteristic of the United States in the last decades, that maximizes individual freedom. Those who staunchly defend Serra start with this premise. But so does the Police Commission in Los Angeles when it agonizes over whether to test an arrested prostitute for infection with the AIDS virus, and so does an Illinois parole board as it tries to assess what to do about a positively tested person who is about to be released and returned to a community that he or she can further infect.

This preoccupation with individualism reflects what is distinctive about the United States. The sense of the individual in American law and society is pervasive and compelling.[7] What Richard Serra vaunts in his sculpture is what we all value: the importance of the citizen, of personal choice, of immunity from the heavy hand of the government. Perhaps this fascination is a veil for self-deceit about the actual amount of autonomy, creativity, and quality of citizenship that we enjoy. But that is a debate for historians. What is clear is that this very emphasis on the individual and autonomy, ersatz or not, may change as a consequence of the AIDS crisis.

Slowly but observably AIDS is already challenging the recently erected legal fortresses that protect the rights of individuals. Laws prohibiting job discrimination have been severely threatened, as teachers who test positive for infection with the AIDS virus are transferred out of classrooms. In a California case, the state's Fair Employment and Housing Commission awarded lost pay to a Raytheon employee who had been removed from his position as quality-control analyst because of an AIDS diagnosis. In Minneapolis, a federal prison inmate who knew he was infected with the AIDS virus was convicted of assault with a deadly weapon for biting two prison guards. The State Department has been sued because of its requirement that all employees and applicants being considered for overseas assignment be tested for infection. Lawyers and psychiatrists are faced with new ethical questions about their duty to disclose information they have confidentially learned about their clients when there is a potential for serious danger to others. Fear of AIDS has become an issue in divorce cases, in child custody proceedings, and on and on.[8]

As the list of legal actions grows longer, the mandate of sustained emergency will inevitably imperil the careful nuances and attention to differences that, thus far, have characterized these court decisions. At some point, the meticulous architecture of rules to ensure that individuals are treated as individuals, not as members of a class, will be jeopardized even more than it normally is. The precise needs and characteristics of particular children, of prospective employees, may be lost in the overwhelming need, the intense fear of the community. That is a hazard we face as we try to ensure the community's survival without sacrificing hard-won individual rights.

The Silent Curriculum of Public Education

During the period of waiting and watching to see how the AIDS epidemic spreads, the emphasis on prevention will intensify. That will mean more of a public commitment to achieving massive changes in personal behavior so as to avoid additional cases of the disease. Oddly, the individual is important as never before. It becomes, in a sense, significantly a matter of individual decision making whether actions are taken that will slow the expansion of the infection. On the other hand, because of the importance of individual choice—and its communal implications—the stage is set for stronger and stronger state intervention. The government will feel compelled to take a wide range of actions, starting with intensive education, to alter the way in which individuality is expressed and to alter our sense of what actions are consistent and inconsistent with cherished notions of freedom.

The debate is no longer over whether there should be sex education in the schools but rather what the nature of that education should be, what signals should be sent, how such education molds or affects personality. As an early step, the AIDS crisis is sure to engender more strength for those who argue that the government can and should constitutionally provide more financial support for parochial schools. The argument will be that these schools—better than public schools—can instill behavioral attitudes that can diminish the spread of AIDS. There are echoes here of previous uses of organized religion as a surrogate, performing some of the roles one might attribute to the state. In the post-Civil War era, for example, Indian reservations were parceled out among major denominations who were given federal financial support to provide a structure and set of principles to fulfill the so-called civilizing mission of the United States.[9]

The declining role of the public schools in shaping conduct is—television and the competition of modern culture aside— the ironic result of the drive to celebrate the individual. The purging of moral content from the public schools arose from a sense that the individual student and the student's family should be free of government-inspired coercion. This philosophy also compelled many who fought to eliminate prayer from the schools, but given the national mood and the composition of the Supreme Court, the likelihood of encouraging moments of silence in the public schools is once again enhanced.[10] The point is not just moments of softly directed silence and the continued modification of Supreme Court decisions. These steps will be taken as a sign that the public schools themselves have more of a job to do in the moral teaching of their students.

In all of these educational matters, the influence of AIDS is now at the margin, but it will move more to the center. Even without the existence of the AIDS crisis, the Governor of New York was pressing for the greater teaching of values in the schools, as was the then-U.S. Secretary of Education, William Bennett. With the AIDS crisis, such instruction will become increasingly compelled, though stripped of much of its moral clothing. Yet any health instruction that deals with sexual conduct is suffused with moral impact, in the view of many parents. When New York City's Health Commissioner first aggressively established television advertisements that counseled safer sex, the Archdiocese and other religious leaders argued that the ads were encouraging casual sexual relations, even though they might be safer ones.

AIDS is the first national text in a great while that even purports to address the propriety of adult behavior. Brochures sent by the government to each household, pamphlets distributed to college students, billboards, public service announcements, newspaper articles, television documentaries, all are part of a pervasive effort to affect the national tone. AIDS becomes a legitimator, sometimes explicitly, sometimes implicitly, for monogamy, constancy, and predictability. It reinstates emotional obstacles to the abrogation of intimate relationships by increasing the cost of achieving new ones. The message of these campaigns is a new focus on what the individual does, not just the heroic individual, or the researcher in the laboratory, but the ordinary person, the parent, the single adult, the adolescent child. All of a sudden, in the national consciousness, what the individual does is meaningful in terms of something larger, something connected to the fate of the community.

Despite the often bitter debate over the specific content of the message to be broadly communicated—the content of public education concerning AIDS—there seems now to be substantial agreement on the essence of the attitudes that must be encouraged: People must know that acts have consequences, that they are responsible for their conduct. The tailored instruction is directed at the phenomenon of AIDS and couched in terms of sexual activity; but the implicit extensions of the message for general conduct are there.

During the early period of AIDS, there were those who defied these changes in personal habits and values, claiming, perhaps rightly by the then-reigning definitions, that sexual activity is the essence of personhood, the essence of individualism. For them, within the messages being communicated to the public about AIDS was a threat to one new-found freedom, the freedom to assert modes of sexual identity. That time of defiance seems to have passed, but the hope exists for a kind of painless accommodation to AIDS, one in which simple precautionary acts, mostly the use of condoms, is all that is required. This is not, according to those who take this perspective, a moment for introspection and radical change but rather a time for minor behavioral reshaping. While there is much to be said for this dissenting view, it is, for the moment, engulfed by the substantial horror of the disease, at least so long as no clear and easy preventive vaccine or cure is available.

For most epidemics in history, what an individual could do had precious little impact on his own health. People fled major urban areas; they wore masks; they tried to avoid public places; they drank to excess; they prayed. None of these individual acts were determinative. Vast changes in sanitation programs, in control of rodents, in development of vaccines—these were the actions that made a substantial impact. At our current level of understanding and scientific expertise in the AIDS crisis, by contrast, control lies far more vith the individual. And because the private and personal conduct of individuals counts so significantly, education and the systematic change of behavior must come from a force more subtle and more powerful than law; coercion is not so successful a strategy.

On the other hand, this programmed propaganda, for that is what it is, must be very carefully considered. In part this is because human sexuality—the conduct at stake—is so basic to our sense of individuality and the concept of freedom in American society. But equally important, we must move cautiously lest the need to educate—suddenly to open windows into the minds and souls of millions—be seen by powerful institutions as a moment for reshaping the American character in its totality, not just as a chance to adjust that character to the needs of the moment. The comprehensive nature of the AIDS crisis has converted almost every form of communication, including advertising and entertainment, into a part of this national educational process. These formidable messages cannot only be about AIDS; they are too forceful and too permeating. At the core of the message being sent out about AIDS is the importance of rethinking the duty of one spouse to another, of lover to lover. This silent curriculum is quietly affecting relationships, though it only rarely requires explicit mention of the reasons for this fundamental change.

The Conundrum of Compassion

The compassion for others that flows from AIDS also has the potential to affect the American character. To be sure, the call is now weak and perhaps temporary. Much of it plays on the need for a privileged "us" to help a removed, separated, and preferably invisible "them." Compassion helps with the project of separation and removal: It can define the harm in such a way that the disease does not belong to the compassionate. AIDS can be another event on a temporary agenda, like sympathy for the Ethiopian famine victims or for the homeless of urban America or for the victims of earthquake in Armenia. That would not be a compassion that sustains a change in the character or actions of the society.

Despite early efforts to make AIDS such a phenomenon, confined to a distinctive group of "others," the sense is now strong that the infection touches us as well as them, that it has the lurking potential to be a societal threat across a wide front. As a consequence, there has been considerable evidence of a growing mood of compassion, in lieu of blame, as a dominant reaction to AIDS. The Gay Men's Health Crisis, one of the leading organizations providing assistance to persons with AIDS, has had so many offers from volunteers that it has had to turn away applicants who wish to help. When the National Institutes of Health established a special facility for AIDS patients, they recruited nurses nationally not by emphasizing wages and working conditions but by appealing to nineteenth-century ideas of service, contribution, and sacrifice.

The AIDS Quarterly, a handsomely produced public television program, which debuted in early 1989, is an example of how themes of compassion and understanding begin to dominate. Peter Jennings, smartly dressed, blue jacket against stark blue background, helps us to fathom AIDS as he helps us to fathom so much else in the world. In its opening segment, "The Education of Admiral Watkins," the program found a proxy for the middle-class viewer of public television and demonstrated how that surrogate becomes more sophisticated, more comprehending. Watkins, reflecting in his packed Washington office, looks out his window on the familiar federal landscape and talks about his evolution as chair of the President's AIDS Commission. Through his mind's eye, we see the shift from AIDS as a gay disease to AIDS as a persistent threat to an underclass he scarcely knew existed. Through him, we have reaffirmed the breakdown in the health care system. Through a recounting of his experiences, we see the children of Harlem Hospital, the bigoted picketing outside schoolyards, the mysterious burning of the house of the young Ray boys in a Florida town—many of the stations in the evolution of our understanding of AIDS.

Watkins becomes a tourguide through changed consciousness, as the military man, stiff and confident, is transformed into the newly comprehending public servant, fearful of the implications of his new knowledge. His is a journey from relative ignorance to deeper understanding, from indifference to anxious concern. He is a convert, depicted, in his origins, as in favor of mandatory testing and at the end seeking to ban any sense of stigma so that a war can be waged against the virus. Watkins is seen as a formerly distant captive of quick and easy answers now forced by circumstances to come to grips with the ties between AIDS and horrific truths of American society. The implication is that this journey is one we all must make.

The powerful final segment of the inaugural *AIDS Quarterly*, entitled "Death in the Family," was even more clearly an essay in compassion. Public television took us to Salt Lake City, Utah, to observe the story of the Pace family, reunited by the dying of their 39-year-old son, Malcolm. We are allowed in, extraordinarily, to observe at length the pain of the deathbed, here not to learn of the sociology of AIDS, nor about its scientific status, but to learn something of its compelling power. This is not about death alone, but death in the family. The metaphor is clear: Every death is a death in the family, our family, the family of mankind.

And the lesson of Malcolm's death is not about the morality of Malcolm's lifestyle; it is turned into a morality play about the need of a son for his father's approval. The stated facts of Malcolm's life are those of a young Mormon boy who violated the faith, who drank, who visited bathhouses, whose loyalty came to be with his "California family," handsome young men with whom Malcolm traveled. These were the facts, but they were not the drama. The fashioners of the story produced not a parable about sexual conduct and blame but one about the dignity and beauty of father–son relations. The episode was romantic in a feeling sense; it was about the way AIDS brought Malcolm's family together, how the father came to appreciate his son and comprehend his own shortcomings. When Malcolm died, virtually before our eyes, two pictures were on the hospital wall: one of his Salt Lake City family, one of his family of friends in California. At the funeral service, his sister speaks of the love of Malcolm for his father, his waiting for his father to come to his bedside before giving way to death. And the final image is a lingering distant perspective of the cemetery, a tiny knot of mourners congregating against the snow-covered mountains of Utah, beneath a sky of brilliant blue.

Some television critics have assaulted the commercial networks for softening the story of AIDS, for avoiding the harshest and rawest of its consequences and emphasizing compassion as a cover for a crueler reality. The charge is that television, more frequently than it shows the agonizing scenes of death and dying of the disdained, presents programs like *Just a Regular Kid*—the story of Ryan White, a typical twelve-year-old boy except that he tests positive for infection with the AIDS virus, a boy full of promise, full of vigor, and hard to place in the standard litany and imagery of AIDS victims. Ryan White came to national prominence because he was barred from his public school. Critics of this television program have charged that by emphasizing the story of this young hero, television producers are diverting attention from the groups at highest risk for AIDS. Since young hemophiliacs with AIDS, like White, can most clearly be defined as innocent, the hidden implication is that the many others who languish in disease are somehow less so.

In the great cities, among the elite, there is room for art shows in which stark photographs of persons with AIDS underscore the ravages of the disease and bring an understanding of its devastation. For the larger society, *Just a Regular Kid* and stories like it are important. We need Ryan White to confirm our sense of the moral fiber of America. Through the retelling of his story, the fear-ridden meaning of AIDS is shifted to an occasion for the celebration of human charity. All AIDS children are pictures of innocence who demand by their very presence that they not be stereotyped, that they not be treated as threats and pariahs. Ryan White is so clearly of the mainstream, a child of Ozzie and Harriet, that he demonstrates how categories become illusory and compassion is required. AIDS becomes a rallying point, a testimony to solidarity. The triumph of Ryan White becomes a tribute to a community that, like Admiral Watkins, started in ignorance but comes to a fuller comprehension of the precise nature of AIDS. The salient image is no longer the bathhouse; it is the huge national quilt of a thousand squares, a flowing monument not to painful death but to personal memories and the victories of friendship.

Here is the side of compassion that is more than a cover for national neglect. Compassion has intense power to alter attitudes, to reduce acts of hostile discrimination, and to provide a hidden defense against the cold conclusions of cost-benefit analysis. Compassion reassures, implying some sense of regained control, well-founded or not.

AIDS is of course more than an American phenomenon, and its calls for compassion extend beyond the towns and cities of the United States. Like other plagues or historically important diseases, it confirms the interrelationship among peoples seemingly distant, geographically and culturally. In earlier times, plague offered a glimpse into the consequences of extensive trading patterns and the complex difficulties of blocking invisible contagion across borders. Then, as now, communities have preferred to believe that disease originated somewhere else, not in their own country, and to define harm as something exterior, confinable to others. The expansion of trade and freedom of movement make the modern world different, in scale if not in kind, from the medieval one. Yet our immediate inclination is also to exclude, to test aliens at the border, to bar visitors from suspect lands. But deep within, the recognition exists that there is no avoiding the interrelatedness of peoples. AIDS confirms our planetary coherence, our inescapable interdependence.

Centuries ago, around Mesa Verde, the brilliant canyons in Colorado, an early people gave up subsistence societies on marginal farmlands and dug themselves, mysteriously, into the sides of cliffs, in strange dwellings, hard to reach, hard to explain. An event of astonishing importance must have led to this substantial change in the place people chose to live their lives. They must have thought they could remove themselves from an enemy, though we do not know whether it was human, spiritual, or environmental threat. In the time of the Black Death, people fled too, finding solace in escape. Today, escape is more difficult because of well-established patterns of cultural interchange, of political and economic interdependence. We could change our patterns of life suddenly and mysteriously, like the people of Mesa Verde. We could try to find the equivalents of cliff dwellings in which to hide. But now, perhaps more than the people of that remote crisis, we sense secretly how temporary such action might be and how unavailing. More realistically, we sense that if the world is to be safe, there cannot be a part of the world, First, Second, or Third, that is the repository of the past history of disease, without the danger that the disease will spring into the present. For that reason alone, we will have a more pragmatic interest in the fate of others, if indeed this interest does not qualify as true compassion.

Protecting Public Health, Preserving Private Life

As was true in Camus' *The Plague,* it is not always the nominal leaders who become the repositories of public trust in a public health emergency. Just as power shifts to military leaders in war, it shifts to the more neutral public health officials during an emergency like AIDS. Society changes because of a desire to have the central issues less vulnerable to the vagaries and injustices of politics. Elected leaders are increasingly perceived as largely the instruments of those in the biomedical establishment who have greater insight into the medical and scientific necessities of the moment. We see it here: an early stage, in which there was a notion that AIDS could be exploited politically, giving way to a period of statesmanship in which virtually no candidate for public office made the issue an important one, despite the deep public concern about it. Finally, it becomes a sullen background event, influencing opinion but not itself a subject of vigorous partisan discourse.

The evolution of the President's AIDS Commission from a collection of people with odd and often irrational biases to a coherent advocate of a deliberate and meaningful national position is an example of the potential for change under duress. As information becomes more and more available, as comprehension increases, approaches that are not reason-based become more hollow-sounding and ineffective, even in motivating emotions and reinforcing political loyalties. And as demands for clear-sightedness, for leadership that depoliticizes grow, there begin to be heroes: Dr. Mathilde Krim, who formed the American Foundation for AIDS Research; the Governor of Indiana, who personally escorted young Ryan White into his school. These are heroes not only in the fight against AIDS but in the fight against prejudice, indifference, and fear. But the emergence of strong leadership willing to provide support for a sustained community approach has not been rapid. A former vice-chair of the President's Commission, a state Health Commissioner who resigned from the Commission early in its history, Woodrow A. Myers, wrote plaintively of the need for "a national consensus on the moral and ethical dimensions of the AIDS epidemic."[11] His call was for a president who would find the courage to discuss the basic issues involved in AIDS, who would encourage trust in public health officials, who would "be our best example of compassion and concern."

It is because of the drastic character of such possible alternatives as quarantines that a public discourse on behavioral change is so important. We can transcend this period of social and political challenge if we can begin to articulate some rules to govern our view of possible public and private actions, find some guidelines designed to acknowledge the existence of a crisis in which public health actions are paramount, while, at the same time, trying to preserve the value we place on individual privacy in a time of stress.

We can, for example, recognize that change in the relationship between the individual and the state is necessary in a time of public health emergency. The great danger is that overreaction and sudden change will take place because of lack of preparation, lack of thought, lack of understanding that the public's health will require modification of much that we know and much that we love about our lives.

We can accept the fact that distinctions may need to be drawn that may have the appearance of discrimination, though a thorough and honest effort must be made to determine whether such distinctions are necessary and reflective of sound judgment. Increasingly, government will have to take actions that would be unthinkable in the absence of the AIDS crisis. The stigmatizing impact of court officials in plastic gloves is an example. In the early stages, there has been more debate about such measures than may be possible if the crisis intensifies. And if it does, there will be less opportunity for time-consuming processes of the sort that were often required for government decisions in the 1970s and 1980s. Providing a forum open to the individual to rail against the clumsy abuses of the state is a hallmark of our system. But the process that is due when dealing with public health issues is less than the process due in criminal proceedings. The question will not be whether new distinctions will be made in such areas as eligibility for private health insurance but how they can be made in the least discriminatory and most rational way.

We can recognize that there is legitimacy to both secular and religious efforts to educate and change personal behavior. Given that there will be some tensions over how society is instructed as to changes in individual behavior, particularly sexual behavior, we will want to encourage organized religion as part of a systematic program to influence the behavior of the young. But we will also want religious organizations to appreciate and encourage the efforts of other private organizations and of government to alter personal behavior, even if implied in their messages is the recognition of conduct not consistent with religious faith.

We can be most sensitive about those areas of law and regulation where the gains have been fragile and reflect hard-fought efforts that could easily be reversed, given the very tenuousness of their current hold on the public. They include the outlawing of employment discrimination, freedom from censorship, the nondiscriminatory right to medical care, the construction of an open system of public education. None of these areas will be immune from regulatory change as a result of AIDS. Indeed, these are the areas where the impact of AIDS is likely to be strongest. But because they are so sensitive, they require particularly careful scrutiny. And, in a public health crisis, this will be difficult.

We must accept that there is to be a greater role for government as a speaker and teacher, though we must be attentive to the dangers in that expanded role. The need for information as a way of dispelling fear, and the need for instruction as part of a general pattern of precaution, is clear. And although much of this task will be carried out through individual action and through the private media, there remains a strong role for government. The question is not whether this should be done—it already is being done—but how and with what principles in mind. In particular, how can information about disease and the necessary precautions be issued without creating an environment that unnecessarily diminishes support for the basic principle of individual rights?

Until technology allows us to approximate a world without AIDS—if that is possible—the state must conduct research, provide treatment, supervise blood supplies, financially support the needy. But it cannot take the actions individuals must take. And that is why a dilemma exists: This is a time for singularly individual responses, but it is also a time in which individual attitudes are being most manipulated by the state and others. If we are fortunate, our private actions, in this moment of community hazard, will fulfill public needs. Failing that, the time may come when the state will, to the extent it thinks possible and consistent with the constitutional interpretations of the moment, seek far more actively to discourage or prevent individuals from conducting themselves in ways that are inimical to the general weal.

Notes

Prologue

1. Richard Goldstein, "Ending AIDS Apartheid," *Village Voice*, December 27, 1987.

2. Michael Durey, *The Return of the Plague: British Society and the Cholera, 1831–1832* (London: Gill and Macmillan, Ltd., 1979), p. 205. See generally William H. McNeill, *Plagues and Peoples* (Garden City, New York: Anchor Press, 1976), the most impressive case for the role of disease in shaping history.

Part One: AIDS and Free Expression

The quotation from Frederick S. Perls is used with the permission of *The Gestalt Journal*.

1. Sexual Imagery and the Media

1. See generally, U.S. House of Representatives, Committee on Education and Labor, *Books for Schools and the Treatment of Minorities* (hearings before the Ad Hoc Subcommittee on De Facto Segregation, 89th Congress, August–September 1966). Frances Fitzgerald, *America Revised: History Schoolbooks in the Twentieth Century* (New York: Vintage Books, 1979), pp. 58–59.

2. Jon Pareles, "Rock's Walk on the Safe Side," *New York Times*, September 20, 1987.

3. Allan Bloom, *The Closing of the American Mind* (New York: Simon and Schuster, 1987), p. 74.

4. Geoffrey Cowan, *See No Evil: The Backstage Battle over Sex and Violence on Television* (New York: Simon and Schuster, 1978), pp. 202–232.

5. 18 United States Code Annotated § 1464 (1984); FCC v. Pacifica Foundation, 438 U.S. 726, 735 (1978), affg. 56 F.C.C. 2d 94 (1975). See also Daniel L. Brenner and Monroe E. Price, *Cable Television and Other Non-broadcast Video* (New York: Clark Boardman and Co., 1986), § 609 [2].

6. The Cable Communications Policy Act of 1984, 47 United States Code § 624 (d)(2)(A); see also Price and Brenner, *Cable Television*, § 609 [3][e]. As broadcasters in an environment of deregulation tolerated more sexually explicit content, advertiser resistance, prodded by audience concern, mounted. See Bill Carter, "TV Sponsors Heed Viewers Who Find Shows Too Racy," *New York Times*, April 23, 1989.

7. Randy Shilts, *And the Band Played On: Politics, People and the AIDS Epidemic* (New York: St. Martin's Press, 1987), pp. 386–387.

8. Simon Watney, *Policing Desire: Pornography, AIDS and the Media* (Minneapolis: University of Minnesota Press, 1987), p. 114.

9. Lucy Kosimar, "The Image of Women in Advertising," in *Women in Sexist Society: Studies in Power and Powerlessness*, ed. Vivian Gornick and Barbara K. Moran (New York: Basic Books, 1971), pp. 306–307. See also Vance Packard, *The Hidden Persuaders* (New York: David McKay, 1957), pp. 84–86.

10. Laurie P. Cohen, "Sex in Ads Becomes Less Explicit, As Firms Turn to Romantic Images," *Wall Street Journal*, Feb. 11, 1988.

11. A. M. Rosenthal, "No Way Out," *New York Times*, Oct. 13, 1987.

12. Similar colloquies between government and the entertainment industry have taken place in which President Bush and others have encouraged voluntary efforts to reduce the glamorization of drug use. For a general discussion of the perilous relationship between the mass media and public discourse, see Neil Postman, *Amusing Ourselves to Death* (New York: Elisabeth Sifton Books, Viking Press, 1985).

2. The Voice of Government in the Marketplace of Ideas

1. Marvin Trachtenberg, *The Statue of Liberty* (New York: Viking Press, 1976), p. 187, and p. 214, n. 11 (quoting from Emma Lazarus, "The New Colossus").

2. Owen Fiss, "Free Speech and Social Structure," *Iowa Law Review*, 71 (1986): 1405, 1410. For a detailed discussion of government speech issues, see S. Shiffrin, "Government Speech," *UCLA Law Review*, 27 (1980): 565.

3. See Action for Children's Television v. FCC, 852 F.2d 1332 (D.C. Cir. 1988). See also Henry John Uscinski, "Deregulating Commercial Television: Will the Marketplace Watch Out for Children?" *American University*

Law Review, 34 (1984): 141–173. See also Matthew L. Spitzer, *Seven Dirty Words and Six Other Stories* (New Haven: Yale University Press, 1986), pp. 95–118, 124–130.

4. Pierce v. Society of Sisters, 268 U.S. 510, 535 (1925).

5. Ibid., p. 534.

6. 262 U.S. 390 (1923).

7. 406 U.S. 205 (1972).

8. See the debate among the Supreme Court Justices in Wallace v. Jaffree, 472 U.S. 38 (1985). Laurence H. Tribe discusses the role of history in constitutional interpretation in his *American Constitutional Law*, 2nd ed. (Mineola, New York: Foundation Press, 1988), pp. 1158–1166. See also Thomas J. Curry, *The First Freedoms: Church and State in America to the Passage of the First Amendment* (New York: Oxford University Press, 1986); Leonard Levy, *The Establishment Clause and the First Amendment* (New York: Macmillan, 1986); Gordon Wood, *Creation of the American Republic, 1776–1787* (Chapel Hill: University of North Carolina Press, 1969), pp. 91–107; for a broader evolutionary span see Morris Janowitz, *The Reconstruction of Patriotism: Education and Civic Consciousness* (Chicago: The University of Chicago Press, 1983), p. 4.

9. Owen Fiss, "Free Speech and Social Structure," *Iowa Law Review*, 71 (1986): 1405, 1409.

10. Mark Yudof, *When Government Speaks: Politics, Law and Government Expression in America* (Berkeley: University of California Press, 1983), p. 57.

11. Ibid., p. 60.

12. Ibid., p. 61.

13. The debate over the Helms amendment is summarized in Josh Getlin, "Attack on 'Safe Sex': Rules Stir AIDS Debate," *Los Angeles Times*, April 28, 1988. For a general discussion of the fracas over methods of prevention through public education, see Ronald Bayer, *Private Acts, Social Consequences* (New York: Free Press, 1989), pp. 207–231.

14. Edwin Meese III, "Memorandum for the Domestic Policy Council," February 11, 1987. The notion of "meaning" has, of course, always been a subject of intense controversy; indeed, there is a veritable interpretation industry among scholars. Some argue that the First Amendment is the embodiment of the enlightenment, a distillation of theory, with only glancing relationship to the social institutions of the day. At the other end of the debate are those for whom social institutions and political interests are the true causative aspects of constitutional meaning. Compare Andrew Reck, "Natural Law and the Constitution, *Review of Metaphysics*, 42 (March

1989): 483, with Charles Beard, *An Economic Interpretation of the Constitution* (New York, 1935). See also R. Weisberg, "Text into Theory: A Literary Approach to the Constitution," *Georgia Law Review*, 20 (1986): 939, and the numerous authorities cited therein.

3. Discrimination at Society's Margin

1. Jew Ho v. Williamson, 103 F. 10, 23, 24 (N.D. Cal. 1890), quoting Yick Wo v. Hopkins, 118 U.S. 356, 373–374 (1886).

2. William Booth, "The Odyssey of a Brochure on AIDS," *Science*, September 18, 1987, p. 237.

3. Ronald Bayer, *Private Acts, Social Consequences: AIDS and the Politics of Public Health* (New York: Free Press, 1989), p. 224.

4. Michael Sanson, "AIDS: A Report for Managers," *Restaurant Management*, May 1987, p. 64.

4. The Vocabulary of Concern

1. Janet (Genet) Flanner, *Paris Journal: 1944–1965* (New York: Atheneum, 1965), p. 7. For the relationship of language to illness, the seminal work remains Susan Sontag's *Illness as Metaphor* (New York: Vintage Books, 1979).

2. 323 U.S. 214 (1944).

3. Ibid., pp. 218, 219, 220.

4. Ibid., pp. 224–225.

5. Ibid., p. 231.

6. 320 U.S. 81, 106, 107 (1943).

7. Richard Goldstein, "Ending AIDS Apartheid," *Village Voice*, December 27, 1987.

8. See Baruch S. Blumberg, "Hepatitis B Virus and the Carrier Problem," *Social Research*, 55 (Autumn 1988): 401.

9. William H. McNeill, *Plagues and Peoples* (Garden City, New York: Anchor Press, 1976), p. 122.

10. Michael Durey, *The Return of the Plague: British Society and the Cholera, 1831–1832* (London: Gill and Macmillan, Ltd., 1979), p. 150.

11. Ibid.

12. David A. J. Richards, "Human Rights, Public Health, and the Idea of Moral Plague," *Social Research*, 55 (Autumn 1988): 491, 526. See also Susan Sontag, *AIDS and Its Metaphors* (New York: Farrar, Straus and Giroux, 1989).

13. United States v. Carolene Products Co., 304 U.S. 144, 153 n.4 at 153 (1938) (referring to Nixon v. Herndon, 286 U.S. 73 (1932).

14. John Hart Ely, *Democracy and Distrust: A Theory of Judicial Review* (Cambridge: Harvard University Press, 1980), p. 153 (quoting Goodman, "De facto School Desegregation: A Constitutional and Empirical Analysis," *California Law Review*, 60 (1972): 275, 313.

15. Ibid., p. 153.

16. 118 U.S. 356 (1886).

17. Ely, *Democracy and Distrust*, p. 162, n. 14.

18. Ronald Bayer, *Private Acts, Social Consequences: AIDS and the Politics of Public Health* (New York: Free Press, 1989), p. 163.

5. Lost Mastery

1. Lewis Thomas, "Science and Health—Possibilities, Probabilities and Limitations," *Social Research*, 55 (Autumn 1988): 379, 394.

2. Douglas Shenson, "When Fear Conquers: A Doctor Learns about AIDS from Leprosy," *New York Times* Magazine, Feb. 28, 1988.

3. Joshua Lederberg, "Pandemic as a Natural Evolutionary Phenomenon," *Social Research*, 55 (Autumn 1988): 343, 347.

4. Ibid., p. 347.

5. Ibid., p. 353.

6. Lewis Thomas, "Science and Health: Possibilities, Probabilities and Limitations," *Social Research*, 55 (Autumn 1988): 379–389.

7. Arien Mack, "In Time of Plague: Five Centuries of Infectious Disease in the Visual Arts," exhibition brochure, American Museum of Natural History, January 1988.

8. Alice Yang, curatorial statement on AIDS exhibition, New Museum, 1989.

6. Searching for a New Paradigm

1. On abortion, see Roe v. Wade, 410 U.S. 113 (1973); on use of contraceptives by married couples, see Griswold v. Connecticut, 381 U.S. 479 (1965); on home reading of obscene materials, see Stanley v. Georgia, 394 U.S. 557 (1969).

2. United States v. Seeger, 380 U.S. 163 (1965). See C.Clancy and J. Weiss, "The Conscientious Objector Exemption: Problems in Conceptual Clarity and Constitutional Considerations," *Maine Law Review*, 17 (1965): 143.

3. Miranda v. Arizona, 384 U.S. 436 (1966).

4. See for example M. Glendon, "Marriage and the State: The Withering Away of Marriage," *Virginia Law Review*, 62 (1969): 663, 703.

5. See for example Richard A. Posner, *The Economics of Justice* (Cambridge: Harvard University Press, 1981).

6. For the artist's account, see Richard Serra " 'Tilted Arc' Destroyed," *Art in America*, 77 (May 1989): 34.

7. See for example Robert N. Bellah et al., *Habits of the Heart: Individualism and Commitment in American Life* (Berkeley: University of California Press, 1985), p. viii.

8. The Intergovernmental Health Project of George Washington University, among others, tracks ever-changing state law and regulation. See also Centers for Disease Control, *Morbidity and Mortality Weekly Report*. For example, see "Partner Notification for Preventing Human Immunodeficiency Virus Infection—Colorado, Idaho, South Carolina, Virginia," *Morbidity and Mortality Weekly Report*, 37, no. 25 (1988): 393–396, 401–402.

9. See Monroe E. Price, *Law and the American Indian* (Indianapolis: Bobbs Merrill, 1973), pp. 693–699; Quick Bear v. Leupp, 210 U.S. 50 (1908).

10. On the relationship between compliance and doctrine in the school prayer context, see Kenneth M. Dolbeare and Phillip E. Hammond, *The School Prayer Decisions* (Chicago: University of Chicago Press, 1971) and W. K. Muir, *Prayers in the Public Schools* (Chicago: University of Chicago Press, 1967).

11. Woodrow A. Myers, Jr., "AIDS: A Presidential Issue," *Wall Street Journal*, December 30, 1987.

Bibliography

Books

Altman, Dennis. *AIDS in the Mind of America*. Garden City, New York: Anchor Press, Doubleday, 1985.

Aries, Phillippe. *Centuries of Childhood: A Social History of Family Life*. Trans. Robert Baldick. New York: Vintage Books, 1962.

Barnouw, Erik. *A Tower of Babel: A History of Broadcasting in the United States*. New York: Oxford University Press, 1966.

Bateson, Mary Catherine, and Richard Goldsby. *Thinking AIDS: The Sociological Response to the Biological Threat*. Reading, Mass.: Addison-Wesley, 1988.

Bayer, Ronald. *Private Acts, Social Consequences: AIDS and the Politics of Public Health*. New York: Free Press, 1989.

Beard, Charles. *An Economic Interpretation of the Constitution*. New York, 1935.

Bellah, Robert N., et al. *Habits of the Heart: Individualism and Commitment in American Life*. Berkeley: University of California Press, 1985.

Bloom, Allan. *The Closing of the American Mind*. New York: Simon & Schuster, 1987.

Bollinger, Lee C. *The Tolerant Society*. New York: Oxford University Press, 1986.

Brandt, Allan M. *No Magic Bullet: A Social History of Venereal Disease in the United States since 1880, "With a New Chapter on AIDS."* New York: Oxford University Press, 1987.

Brenner, Daniel L., and Monroe E. Price. *Cable Television and Other Nonbroadcast Video*. New York: Clark Boardman and Co., 1986.

Buchdal, G. *Metaphysics and the Philosophy of Science. The Classic Origins: Descartes to Kant*. Oxford: Oxford University Press, 1963.

Camus, Albert. *The Plague*. New York: Vintage Books, 1972.

Cochrane, A. L. *Effectiveness and Efficiency: Random Reflections on Health Services*. London: Oxford University Press, 1972.

Cowan, Geoffrey. *See No Evil: The Backstage Battle over Sex and Violence on Television*. New York: Simon and Schuster, 1978.

Crosby, Alfred W., Jr. *Epidemic and Peace, 1918*. Connecticut: Greenwood Press, 1976.

Curry, Thomas J. *The First Freedoms: Church and State in America to the Passage of the First Amendment*. New York: Oxford University Press, 1986.

Dalton, Harlan. *AIDS and the Law: A Guide for the Public*. New Haven: Yale University Press, 1987.

D'Emilio, John, and Estelle B. Freedman. *Intimate Matters: A History of Sexuality in America*. New York: Harper & Row, 1988.

Diggins, John P. *The Lost Soul of American Politics: Virtue, Self-Interest, and the Foundations of Liberalism*. Chicago: University of Chicago Press, 1984.

Dijesterhuis, E. *The Mechanisation of the World Picture*. London: Oxford University Press, 1961.

Dolbeare, Kenneth M., and Phillip E. Hammond. *The School Prayer Decisions*. Chicago: University of Chicago Press, 1971.

Dreuilhe, Emmanuel. *Mortal Embrace*. Trans. Linda Coverdale. New York: Hill and Wang, 1988.

Dubos, R. *Man, Medicine, Environment*. New York: Mentor, 1968.

Durey, Michael. *The Return of the Plague: British Society and the Cholera, 1831–1832*. London: Gill and Macmillan, Ltd., 1979.

Ely, John Hart. *Democracy and Distrust: A Theory of Judicial Review*. Cambridge: Harvard University Press, 1980.

Erikson, Erik H. *Identity: Youth and Crisis*. New York: W. W. Norton, 1968.

Fee, Elizabeth, and Daniel M. Fox. *AIDS: The Burdens of History*. Berkeley: University of California Press, 1988.

Fellman, Anita Clair, and Michael Fellman. *Making Sense of Self: Medical Advice Literature in Late 19th Century America*. Philadelphia: University of Pennsylvania Press, 1981.

Firth, Simon, ed. *Facing the Music*. New York: Pantheon Books, 1988.

Fitzgerald, Frances. *America Revised: History Schoolbooks in the Twentieth Century*. New York: Vintage Books, 1979.

Flanner, Janet. *Paris Journal: 1944–1965*. New York: Atheneum, 1965.

Foucault, Michel. *The Birth of the Clinic*. London: Tavistock Press, 1973.

Gasquet, Francis Aidan. *The Black Death of 1348 and 1349*. London: George Bell and Sons, 1908.

Gilman, Sander L. *Disease and Representation: Images of Illness from Madness to AIDS*. Ithaca: Cornell University Press, 1988.

Glick, Paul C. *American Families*. New York: John Wiley and Sons, 1957.

Goffman, Erving. *Gender Advertisements*. Cambridge: Harvard University Press, 1979.

Gornick, Vivian, and Barbara K. Moran, eds. *Women in Sexist Society: Studies in Power and Powerlessness*. New York: Basic Books, 1971.

Gottfried, Robert S. *The Black Death: Natural and Human Death in Medieval Europe*. New York: Free Press, 1983.

Harris, Marvin. *America Now: The Anthropology of a Changing Culture*. New York: Simon and Schuster, 1981.

Herzlich, Claudine, and Jannine Pierret. *Illness and Self in Society*. Trans. Elborg Forster. Baltimore: Johns Hopkins University Press, 1984.

Illich, Ivan. *Medical Nemesis: The Expropriation of Health*. New York: Pantheon Books, 1976.

Janowitz, Morris. *The Reconstruction of Patriotism: Education for Civic Consciousness*. Chicago: University of Chicago Press, 1983.

Kleiman, Mark A. R. *AIDS, Vice and Public Policy: Working Paper*. Cambridge, Mass.: John F. Kennedy School of Government, 1987.

Konvitz, Milton R. *Religious Liberty and Conscience: A Constitutional Inquiry*. New York: Viking Press, 1968.

Kurland, Philip B. *Religion and the Law: Of Church and State and the Supreme Court*. Chicago: Aldine Publishing Co., 1962.

Leavitt, Judith Walzer, and Ronald L. Numbers. *Sickness and Health in America*. Madison: University of Wisconsin Press, 1985.

Leites, Edmund. *The Puritan Conscience and Modern Sexuality*. New Haven: Yale University Press, 1986.

Levy, Leonard W. *Emergence of a Free Press*. New York: Oxford University Press, 1985.

——*The Establishment Clause and the First Amendment*. New York: Macmillan, 1986.

Link, Vernon B. *A History of Plague in the United States*. Washington, D.C.: U.S. Department of Health, Education and Welfare, Public Health Department, 1955.

MacKinnon, Catharine A. *Feminism Unmodified: Discourses on Life and Law*. Cambridge, Mass.: Harvard University Press, 1987.

Manzoni, Alessandro. *I the Betrothed*. London: Aldine Press, 1951.

Masters, William H., Virginia E. Johnson, and Robert C. Kolodny. *Crisis: Heterosexual Behavior in the Age of AIDS*. New York: Grove Press, 1988.

McNeill, William H. *Plagues and Peoples*. Garden City, New York: Anchor Press, 1976.

Mead, Margaret. *Culture and Commitment: A Study of the Generation Gap*. Garden City, New York: Natural History Press, 1970.

Merelman, Richard M. *Making Something of Ourselves: On Culture and Politics in the United States.* Berkeley: University of California Press, 1984.

Montgomery, Kathryn C. *Target: Prime Time: Advocacy Groups and the Struggle over Entertainment Television.* New York: Oxford University Press, 1989.

Muir, W. K. *Prayer in the Public Schools.* Chicago: University of Chicago Press, 1967.

Navarro, V. *Medicine under Capitalism.* New York: Prodist, 1976.

Nelkin, Dorothy. *Selling Science: How the Press Covers Science and Technology.* New York: W. H. Freeman and Co., 1987.

Neustadt, Richard E., and Ernest R. May. *Thinking in Time: The Uses of History for Decision Makers.* New York: Free Press, 1986.

Osborne, June, ed. *History, Science and Politics: Influenza in America 1918–1976.* New York: Prodist, 1977.

Packard, Vance. *The Hidden Persuaders.* New York: David McKay, 1957.

Panem, Sandra. *The AIDS Bureaucracy.* Cambridge: Harvard University Press, 1988.

Pattison, Robert. *The Triumph of Vulgarity: Rock Music in the Mirror of Romanticism.* New York: Oxford University Press, 1987.

Pierce, Christin, and Donald VanDeVeer. *AIDS: Ethics and Public Policy.* Belmont, Calif.: Wadsworth Publishing Company, 1988.

Posner, Richard A. *The Economics of Justice.* Cambridge: Harvard University Press, 1981.

Postman, Neil. *Amusing Ourselves to Death: Public Discourse in the Age of Show Business.* New York: Elisabeth Sifton Books, Viking Press, 1985.

Powe, Lucas A., Jr. *American Broadcasting and the First Amendment.* Berkeley: University of California Press, 1987.

Price, Monroe E. *Law and the American Indian.* Indianapolis: Bobbs Merrill, 1973.

Rosen, G. *From Medical Police to Social Medicine: Essays on the History of Health.* New York: Science History Publications, 1974.

Rosen, Marjorie. *Popcorn Venus.* New York: Avon, 1974.

Rosenberg, Charles E. *The Cholera Years.* Chicago: University of Chicago Press, 1987.

Schur, Edwin M. *The Americanization of Sex.* Philadelphia: Temple University Press, 1988.

Shilts, Randy. *And the Band Played On: Politics, People and the AIDS Epidemic.* New York: St. Martin's Press, 1987.

Shyrock, R. *The Development of Modern Medicine.* New York: Hafner, 1969.

Sontag, Susan. *AIDS and Its Metaphors.* New York: Farrar, Straus and Giroux, 1989.

—— *Illness as Metaphor.* New York: Vintage Books, 1979.

Spitzer, Matthew L. *Seven Dirty Words and Six Other Stories.* New Haven: Yale University Press, 1986.

Starr, Paul. *The Social Transformation of American Medicine.* New York: Basic Books, 1982.

Trachtenberg, Marvin. *The Statue of Liberty.* New York: Viking Press, 1976.

Tribe, Laurence H. *American Constitutional Law.* 2nd ed. Mineola, New York: Foundation Press, 1988.

Tussman, Joseph. *Government and the Mind.* New York: Oxford University Press, 1977.

Watney, Simon. *Policing Desire: Pornography, AIDS and the Media.* Minneapolis: University of Minnesota Press, 1987.

Williamson, Judith. *Consuming Passions: The Dynamics of Popular Culture.* London: Marion Boyars, 1987.

Wood, Gordon. *Creation of the American Republic, 1776–1787.* Chapel Hill: University of North Carolina Press, 1969.

Yudof, Mark G. *When Government Speaks: Politics, Law and Government Expression in America.* Berkeley: University of California Press, 1983.

Ziegler, Philip. *The Black Death.* Torchbooks: New York, 1969.

Scholarly Articles, Symposia, Reports, and Other Publications

From among the thoughtful symposia that were of benefit in preparing this study, I would single out one called "In Times of Plague: The History and Social Consequences of Epidemic Disease," held at the New School in January 1988 (published in *Social Research,* vol. 55, no. 3). *Medicine and Health Care,* 14 (1988) contains a thoughtful series of essays, edited by L. Gortin and W. J. Curran, on "AIDS, Science and Epidemiology." *October,* vol. 43 (1987), is devoted to "AIDS: Cultural Analysis, Cultural Activism," edited by Douglas Crimp. The Milbank Memorial Fund has published one special issue dealing with AIDS, "AIDS: The Public Context of an Epidemic," *Milbank Quarterly,* vol. 64, supplement 1 (1986). Another issue, with a stellar roster, is scheduled for publication in late 1989. A special issue of *Daedalus,* vol. 118, no. 2, "Living with AIDS," contains a number of significant essays.

The daily accounts in the *New York Times, Newsday,* the *Wall Street Journal,* and the *Los Angeles Times,* as well as weekly reports in the *Village Voice, Time, Newsweek,* and other publications, were vital to the research for this book. The essays of Richard Goldstein in the *Village Voice* were particularly helpful.

AIDS: Public Policy Dimensions. New York: United Hospital Fund and the Institute for Health Policy Studies, 1987.

Arras, John D. "The Fragile Web of Responsibility: AIDS and the Duty to Treat." *Hastings Center Report,* April/May 1988, pp. 10–20.

Blumberg, Baruch S. "Hepatitis B Virus and the Carrier Problem." *Social Research,* 55 (Autumn 1988): 401–412.

Booth, William. "The Odyssey of a Brochure on AIDS." *Science,* September 18, 1987, p. 237.

Clancy, C., and J. Weiss. "The Conscientious Objector Exemption." *Maine Law Review,* 17 (1965): 143–160.

Crimp, Douglas. "AIDS: Cultural Analysis, Cultural Activism." *October,* 43 (1987): 3–16.

Eisenberg, Leon. "The Genesis of Fear: AIDS and the Public's Response to Science." *Law, Medicine and Health Care: AIDS, Science and Epidemiology,* 14, nos. 5–6 (December 1986): 243–249.

Figlio, K. "The Historiography of Scientific Medicine: An Invitation to the Human Sciences." *Comparative Studies in Society and History,* 19 (1977): 262–286.

Fiss, Owen. "Free Speech and Social Structure." *Iowa Law Review,* 71 (1986): 1405–1425.

Glendon, M. "Marriage and the State." *Virginia Law Review,* 62 (1969): 663–720.

Gould, Robert. "AIDS: A Doctor Tells Who May Not Be at Risk." *Cosmopolitan,* January 1, 1988.

Hammet, Theodore M. *AIDS in Correctional Facilities: Issues and Options.* Washington, D.C.: U.S. Department of Justice, National Institute of Justice, 1988. 3rd ed.

Institute of Medicine and National Academy of Science. *Confronting AIDS.* Washington, D.C.: National Academy Press, 1986.

Jewson, N. "The Disappearance of the Sick Man from Medical Cosmology: 1770–1870." *Sociology,* 10, no. 2 (1976): 225–244.

Lederberg, Joshua. "Pandemic as a Natural Evolutionary Phenomenon." *Social Research,* 55, no. 3 (Autumn 1988): 343–359.

New York Commission on Human Rights. *AIDS and People of Color: The Discriminatory Impact.* New York: August 1987.

Office of Technology Assessment, Congress of the United States. *AIDS and Health Insurance.* Staff Paper 2. Washington, D.C.: U.S. Printing Office, February 1988.

―――― *How Effective Is AIDS Education?* Staff Paper 3. Washington, D.C.: U.S. Printing Office, June 1988.

—— *Review of the Public Health Response to AIDS: A Technical Memorandum.* Washington, D.C.: U.S. Printing Office, February 1985.

Report of the Presidential Commission on the Human Immunodeficiency Virus Epidemic. 0-214-701. Washington, D.C.: U.S. Printing Office, 1988. (Popularly known as the "Report of the President's AIDS Commission.")

Reck, Andrew. "Natural Law and the Constitution." *Review of Metaphysics,* 42 (March 1989): 483–512.

Ribicoff, A., and P. Deacan. *The American Medical Machine.* New York: Saturday Review Press, 1972.

Richards, David A. J. "Human Rights, Public Health and the Idea of Moral Plague." *Social Research,* 55, no. 3 (Autumn 1988): 491–528.

Serra, Richard. " 'Tilted Arc' Destroyed." *Art in America,* 77 (May 1989): 34–47.

Shiffrin, S. "Government Speech." *UCLA Law Review,* 27 (1980): 565.

Thomas, Lewis. "Science and Health: Possibilities, Probabilities, and Limitations." *Social Research,* 55, no. 3 (Autumn 1988): 379–395.

Uscinski, Henry John. "Deregulating Commercial Television." *American University Law Review* 34 (1984): 141–173.

Weisberg, R. "Text into Theory: A Literary Approach to the Constitution." *Georgia Law Review,* 20 (1986): 939–994.

Willis, David P., Ronald Bayer, and Daniel M. Fox, eds. "AIDS: The Public Context of an Epidemic." *Milbank Quarterly,* 64, supplement 1 (1986).

Acknowledgments

Despite the brevity of this work, I have many people to thank. David and Lucy Eisenberg and Bettyann Kevles said and did the right things at the necessary times to assure that the project would continue. A summer at the Shaker Mill Inn near New Lebanon, New York—its congenial mood established by Ingram Papernay—permitted me to begin the writing. Susan Wallace was a kind, wise, and forceful editor. Howard Boyer and Nikki Smith merged imagination and commerce in finding a home for the book. Ronald Bayer, Robert Burt, Edward de Grazia, Shepard Forman, Kathy Kudlick, Richard Kurnit, Tom Laqueur, David Michaels, Sheldon Nodelman, Paul Shupack, Grant Ujifusa, and Jonathan Weiss read and commented on parts of the manuscript.

I am grateful to the Jacob Burns Institute for Advanced Legal Studies and to my colleagues at Yeshiva University's Benjamin N. Cardozo School of Law for their dedication to ideas. Their spirit of inquiry nourished this work and permitted me to see the writing of this book as part of my duties as dean. Lisa Thurau, as my principal research assistant, brought passion, patience, and insight to the project. Peter Brooks, Amy Faust, Laura Markham, Julie Price, Betty Rothbart, and Susan Tucker also helped me with the research, as did Lynn Wishart, Norma Feld, Mary Thompson, and the loyal staff of the Cardozo Library. Millie Morgan painstakingly prepared the manuscript. Aimée Brown Price provided a critical eye, her high standard of scholarship as a model, and, when needed, encouragement and solace.

Index